Just Have Sex

An Infertility Memoir

A. L. Guion

LIBRA LIBROS LLC

Libra Libros LLC

CONTENTS

Copyright   V

Dedication   VI

Epigraph   VII

Acknowledgments   VIII

Introduction   X

1. Chapter 1   1

2. Chapter 2   8

3. Chapter 3   11

4. Chapter 4   21

5. Chapter 5   30

6. Chapter 6   39

7. Chapter 7   48

8. Chapter 8   57

9. Chapter 9   64

10. Chapter 10   71

11. Chapter 11   86

12. Chapter 12   100

13. Chapter 13   106

14. Chapter 14   116

15. Chapter 15   125

16. Chapter 16   133

17. Chapter 17   142

18. Chapter 18   146

19. Chapter 19   156

20. Chapter 20   163

21. Chapter 21   174

22. Chapter 22   187

23. Chapter 23   195

24. Chapter 24   202

25. Chapter 25   216

Timeline   228

About the Author   230

Other books by A. L. Guion   232

Cheat Sheet for well-meaning but irritating friends and   234
family

WARNING: THIS BOOK DEALS WITH SENSITIVE CONTENT SUCH AS PREGNANCY, PREGNANCY LOSS, INFERTILITY, AND INFREQUENT BUT PRESENT SWEARING. IF THAT'S NOT YOUR CUP OF TEA... *BACK AWAY SLOWLY*.

Though this is a story of our experience, some is a work of fiction. Names, characters, places, and incidents are either the product of the author's imagination or are used fictitiously.

Some names and places have been changed to protect privacy. Any resemblance to actual persons, living or dead, events, or locales is entirely coincidental. Experiences and dialogue vary but I did my best to recount them to the best of my memory (or to boil them down for readability). As is life, participants have different versions of what they experienced, but these events are remembered and recounted here by how they affected me. The impact on my journey and psyche during this time cannot be argued, though the dialogue or other person's intent may be.

Dedication

This book is dedicated to my husband, Josh.
embryo miracle, Cooper; surprise miracle, Owen.

And to all who may need it: I hope that this sharing enlightens, encourages,
and inspires.

We Plan, God laughs

– Yiddish Proverb (I think :-))

ACKNOWLEDGMENTS

This book wouldn't have been possible without Josh. Not only because he was the other half of our embryo sandwich but because he encouraged me to share our story to help others. If this book can help just one person navigate the iceberg of infertility, then I consider it a success. **Thank you, Josh**, for rewatching our old videos, reading through our old notes, reminiscing on that very difficult time, proofreading, and for being so supportive of me writing this book during naps and after bedtimes. My head might always be one million miles away, but my heart's *always* with you and the kids.

Thank you to my parents for dealing with my craziness and sometimes rather depressing attitude during this extremely challenging time. **Thank you, Dad**, for being steadfast and unflappable. Listening quietly and never casting judgment. **Thank you, Mom**, for loving me anyways, even when I was awful to you. You're the bestest bestie in the whole world, and thanks for not holding my awfulness against me. **Thank you both for supporting us in this journey (in all the ways you both know you did).**

Thank you, friends (you know who you are), for still loving me even when I went heartsore for a little while. Attending your kids' one-year birthday parties or gender reveals was a unique kind of torture, and I was grieving and depressed. Thank you for sticking by me anyways. I'm better now :-)

And ***thank you, dear reader***, for taking a chance on this book. As you follow our journey, I hope you'll learn just how 'not alone' you really are. Every journey is different. Be easy on yourself and try not to compare. But if you were like me, you might find comfort in reading about someone else who battled the titans of infertility. We may be few, but we are strong. Wherever your journey leads, only *you* can decide when it's over. Take heart and do what is best for you.

(ALSO, I'M NOT A MEDICAL PROFESSIONAL, DON'T TAKE ANY OF MY NOVEL AS MEDICAL ADVICE!)

Introduction

You know that dream? The one where you grow up and fall in love with someone who thinks you walk on water. You then get married, have two point four kids, a nice house with a white picket fence, and a Golden Retriever (or, in my case, a German Shepherd).

I always thought my life was right on track for that. I had an *amazing* childhood. My parents were arguably the best parents ever. I sat next to this freshman superstar in Spanish class while I was in the ninth grade, who thought I was pretty cool. We dated throughout high school. We dated throughout college. We both got great jobs out of college. We got married. We got a house on a dead-end road, only a couple miles away from my childhood home in a small southern New Hampshire town. And though it didn't have a white picket fence, we had our German Shepherd, and our life was pretty perfect. But an ominous dark cloud was casting a shadow on our otherwise perfect life. We were told we couldn't have kids (at least not naturally).

We struggled for three years to get answers, and we finally received them. IVF was our only option. And throughout that journey, I was an emotional train wreck. You name the emotion, and believe me, I experienced it.

I grew up in a town where if you didn't have a husband by nineteen and a baby by twenty-one, then you would clearly die alone (see Kacey Musgraves 'Merry-Go-Round'). At a time when all my cousins and friends were pro-creating and experiencing the ups and downs of parenting, my husband and I could only watch, wish, and wait.

We decided to write about our journey. To tell our story. To reach out to people like us who were also struggling and had no idea what the future would hold. I'm not a super religious person, but I have come to appreciate the phrase "you make plans, and God laughs."

My husband and I frequently joke that the hilarity of our life, situations, and experiences are straight out of a sitcom. We even have a running gag that I'll look towards our "studio audience" off to the side when he does something ridiculous. "If only we could have had that on tape" is a commonly used phrase (however outdated it may be).

This book is part of our story, though somewhat fictionalized for better reading (we'll let you wonder what parts were made up. A hint: not many). Hopefully, you will find comfort in not being alone because you are not alone by any means. I want you to see the silver lining in the dark and gloomy clouds surrounding you. Believe me, "it's worth every heartache."

(And, because it warrants mentioning twice, I'm not a medical professional, don't take ANY of my novel as medical advice!)

One

"So, when are you going to have a baby?"

I smiled and laughed as I answered the question for the tenth time that night. "We're going to pay down some debt first. Then we'll be all about those babies!" I gushed to my aunt and lifted my champagne flute to my lips, smiling indulgently. My mom bought us a pair of matching Waterford Crystal flutes for the wedding, and they matched the purple sash of my dress perfectly. She was my Matron of Honor, and she tackled wedding planning with an enthusiasm that beat even my own. With her help, everything was going as planned. Everything was perfect.

Sort of like my life in general.

I looked out over the guests, eating, mingling, drinking, and dancing, and sought my husband. He was on his 'side' of the reception hall. Our families had little in common, discounting that we were all humans, alive, on planet Earth. As such, we split the families down the middle of the aisle. Mine to the right, his to the left. However, the two families did have one thing in common, besides us glowing newlyweds. His mother's parents had adopted a few of their kids, and my mother's parents adopted all of their kids. So, we both had adopted aunts and uncles that we grew up with. Not enough of a conversation piece to bond about during Christmas dinners... or weddings. I smiled benignly at a passing relative and moved toward my new hubby.

Naturally, when I got to him, I heard the gentle clinking and clanking of silverware on glassware, so we leaned in for our customary kiss.

The kiss was as familiar as breathing. I knew exactly what flavor gum I'd taste. I knew exactly how my husband would tilt his head. I knew exactly where he'd place his hand on my waist. It was home.

We spent the next few hours catching up with family and friends and just having a really expensive party. We posed for the camera, danced to our favorite songs, and serenaded each other to ridiculous songs that the DJ played. Instinctively, when "Don't Stop Believing" (a requirement of practically every wedding ever) came on, we grabbed each other dramatically and yelled the lyrics at the top of our lungs. The song's message was lost in the night's energy, but I should have paid more attention.

The day was perfect. Everything went according to plan, and life was wonderful. Time stood still, if only for that one day. There was no drama, no struggles, no family obligations. Instead, it was about us and the future we would create together. We have worked towards this for nine years, and we'd accomplish even more in the next nine. And the nine after that. And the nine after that.

The world was our oyster. We could shape it however we wanted. We worked hard to set ourselves up for success - in whatever capacity that was.

And nothing was going to stop us.

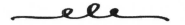

"Josh, will you come here and help me pull these pins out?" I called from the bathroom as I tried to undo the complicated updo. I slammed my hands on the countertop in frustration.

Josh entered the bathroom, half undressed out of his grey suit and looked at my hair. Just a couple inches taller than me, he had a direct shot into the back of my head, but not necessarily the top.

"Ashley Lynn." The horror in his voice made me laugh. "What do I even do?"

"Find the bobby-pins holding my hair in place and pull. Gently!" I squealed when he went whole hog on my poor head. Having my hair pinned in place for twelve hours left my scalp tender and bruised. He slowly started picking through the rat's nest. As chunks fell, I used my hands to massage my head and double-check for any lingering bobby pins. There were some casualties of war as strands of my brownish hair were lost in the process. Is pain beauty? I think I had heard that a time or two. I watched the strands clump together in the sink while continuing to trail my hands in the paths that Josh had just cleared. Luckily my hair wasn't incredibly long, just a couple of inches below my shoulders, but even so, it could still get pretty knotted when it wanted to.

I heard the door open downstairs as we worked silently. Though the moon reflected through the window onto our bathroom mirror, sunrise was only a couple of hours away, and I didn't panic. I just figured it was his dad coming to pick us up and take us to the airport for the honeymoon. Living in a quiet town had its advantages; things would be much different in a city.

"How do they think of these things?" Josh mumbled to himself as he pulled more out. "Little torture devices. Makes me glad to be bald."

And indeed, he was. He started going bald when we were fifteen. He bravely fought it, but the ravages of time caught up to him a little more each year. His haircuts became closer and closer to his head until we were about nineteen, and then he started having me buzz his hair without a guide on the end. By the time we were twenty-three, the hair on the top was mostly non-existent, but he managed some soft peach fuzz on the side by his ears. The bald on-top look gave him heebie-jeebies, so he used his shaving razor this past year to shave it all. Bald was a good look for him. My personal Bruce Willis.

Josh and I met in seventh grade. I schemed and plotted ways to get him to notice my best friend and to go out with her. I didn't understand the appeal and thought he was obnoxious.

By the time ninth grade came around, I was just the girl that constantly harassed him about going on a date with my friend, and he was just the guy that repeatedly said no. We had no fond feelings or friendship and no other interactions to build a friendly acquaintance.

However, ninth grade found us with three classes in common. So, we had to get friendly pretty quick. Our first class together was English, with the best teacher ever; she was invited to our wedding many years later. The second class was a study hall - which was a note-passing session for him and a homework session for me. And the third fated class was Spanish II.

We were fresh-eyed ninth graders in a class that boasted all upper-level students. Only a couple of ninth-graders were in that class, so we had to stick together—strength in numbers and all that. Well, as time would show, our teacher had a biting sense of humor and used his fluency in Spanish to roast the upperclassmen that were in the class but not paying attention. And, as luck would have it, both Josh and I had a knack for Spanish. So, we sat there in the corner of our room, us against them, smiling and snickering while our teacher razzed and teased our fellow students. The shared understanding built a bond that spread across the other common classes. We started taking study hall seats near each other, helping each other with homework, and talking about life and sports. Our study hall period was the last of the day, and as we were both freshmen on varsity fall teams, they frequently released us early for games. Again, another thing we could bond over—he was one of two freshmen on the starting varsity soccer squad, and I was one of two on the starting field hockey team. Maybe we had more in common than we had originally thought. I associated him with seventh-grade science class when our teacher was trying to normalize the word 'penis,' and Josh decided it would be funny to shout 'penis' and 'vagina' in class. For a girl who enjoyed being lost in books, the whole thing made my cheeks flame and my eyes roll.

Over the next few years in high school, we were inseparable. We orchestrated our classes to match, which resulted in Josh taking classes that were more work than he wanted to commit to (even though he's the smarter one, just lazier). We had similar interests in sports and movies, and the rest we learned. I introduced him to country music (gasp! It's not all Achy Breaky Heart!), and he introduced me to Lupe Fiasco and Dave Mathews Band. I taught him about field hockey; he taught me about lacrosse. He tried to convince me that vanilla ice cream reigned supreme. I still disagree—chocolate forever.

Our first date was mini-golfing and pizza, and I remember him stopping on the side of the road as we walked there (only fifteen years old, remember?) and picking a flower from the side of the road. I still have that flower somewhere.

Of course, we were hormonal, hot-mess teenagers, so we had our share of angst and drama, but life was pretty great.

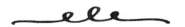

"Hello?" I heard his dad call from downstairs as Josh finished up with the rest of my bobby pins. I ran my hand through my hair to loosen everything up and cringed. Stinky, sweaty, with random hard parts from the hair spray. Decision made; I'd just jump in the shower immediately. Josh could entertain his dad.

"Be right down!" Josh yelled back as I turned on the shower. I had him unzip the top part of my wedding dress and let the rest fall.

"For my next wedding, I'm wearing Spanx, or at least sliding shorts under my dress to prevent chafing," I grumbled to Josh.

"Do you own Spanx?" Josh asked, dead serious.

I didn't. But I would buy some if I needed to.

It was an unseasonably hot day in September. It hit ninety degrees during the middle of our ceremony. After the wedding, I went into the nearest barn, hiked up my skirts, and started fanning myself to let my legs breathe. We didn't mean for the ceremony to take as long as it had, but our officiant read slower than we intended. So, there we were, stuck in the blazing sun. We were suffering right along with our guests. It cooled off as the day progressed, but I was still thankful one of my bridesmaids remembered to pack some deodorant to travel with us.

Josh headed downstairs while I jumped in the shower. I massaged my poor scalp, scrubbed the layers of makeup off my face, and rubbed my aching feet. I felt more human when I got out, but now I was ready for a nap. I was sure that the ever-present dark circles under my hazel eyes were blacker than usual. It was approaching two in the morning, and we still had a long way to go before settling down for a nice, long, restorative sleep.

I vigorously dried my thick hair with the towel as I heard Josh and his dad mumbling from downstairs. They were probably discussing the day and everything that happened. I sighed wistfully. It was picture-perfect. There was its share of dramas—like any wedding—but I wouldn't have changed it for the world. As I brushed my teeth over the sink, I stared at my face in the mirror, amazed at my transformation for the day. I was, simply put, quite ordinary. I boasted light brown hair that developed a blonde tinge in the summer when my hair wasn't drenched from the shower—unimpressive thin lips, a petite nose, and a tall forehead. My chin was pointier than I would prefer, but my two favorite features were my teeth and eyes. My eyes matched my dad's eyes. They are a unique form of hazel that would vary on the day. Some days they were more green, others closer to a light brown, and some days, like today, they were almost topaz. What they were not was blue. Despite what one eye doctor told me once, I didn't end up going back to that quack.

I imagined what our children might look like one day. Would they get my eyes or Josh's eyes? Would they be bald like him (sorry daughters!) or have my thick hair? Would they be of average height like the both of us, or get some gene from one of our parents that made them taller or shorter? I know that I told everyone at the wedding that we would pay down some debt first. And we would. But I had plans. I had dreams. If there was one thing certain in life, it was that I was made to be a mom.

I knew I wanted to be a mom when I was nine years old. I had forgotten a homework assignment that was on one of those big poster boards, and I remember crying as I walked to the front desk. I was so worried that I was going to fail my presentation. The high-strung Type A in me was overreacting and feeling *all-the-feels*, per usual. Now that I reflect on it, there's no way the teacher would have failed me for that. But I called my mom, completely distraught, and she reined me in. She brought it to me, and I passed with flying colors. Crisis averted—Super Mom to the rescue.

And so it went.

My mom saved my butt countless times over the years. From forgetting homework, to actually helping me do my homework, she was my hero. She always had time for me and always knew how to save me from myself. I knew I wanted to be just like her when I grew up. Each school year had a breaking point for me, where I placed so much pressure on myself that I would teeter toward a breakdown. My mom saw those coming from a mile away and would try to bribe me to stay home so I could hang out with her and decompress. Did I mention she was the coolest mom in the world?

She is.

And I knew that I wanted to be just like her (it helped that my dad was pretty amazing too).

I'd pass on the love and awesomeness to my own kids because I learned from the best.

So, Josh and I had plans to pay down debt... but they were rather accelerated and aggressive plans. Because even if his life's purpose wasn't necessarily to be a dad - he still wanted kids (almost) as much as I did.

Two

I HAD A WHOLE chapter devoted to our honeymoon in my original publication. I described our resort, some excursions, and gave you a glimpse into Josh's and my dynamic.

I showed you how Josh was always moving and jittering. The amount of energy he had rivals a two-year-old right when you tell them it's bedtime.

I told you how being prepared and informed was my middle name. Right next to 'always late.'

I let you know that I stopped The Pill when we got engaged because I heard prolonged use could make it hard to get pregnant. Therefore, our only line of defense was condoms. But, as Josh said at the time, "if something gets past the goalie and you get pregnant, that's fine. If not, that's fine too. We have time. I'm not in any rush." Famous last words.

And finally, I described us meeting a couple who opened my eyes to a lot of pregnancy, birth, infertility, and motherhood preconceptions.

Those all-too-common presumptions and frequently uttered judgments haunted me every time I saw another negative pregnancy test or stuck yet another IVF needle in my belly

Ultimately, the original chapter hammered home that people can be opinionated. People can believe their pregnancy and birth plans are the only correct ways to gestate and birth. Some believe that pain meds during delivery are akin to child abuse and the epitome of all selfishness. Some believe that women's bodies are MADE to get pregnant, so no one ever needs to worry about conceiving. And, if you did have trouble conceiving, you either did it to yourself, or you didn't deserve a kid. Boom, 'God's plan.'

Yeah...

Those sentiments haunted me for years during my infertility testing and treatments. For years, I let that poison color my own mind and make me doubt myself. But now? Now, I'm making the executive decision to remove the original chapter from my novel. As such, I've replaced it with this summary chapter that will serve as a reminder to myself, and others, to not let other people corrupt and sully our mental state.

However, this chapter served as a perfect reminder that people usually think their way is best. What I needed to learn over the course of my infertility journey was that there are very few times in life when there is only 'one' right way. As my family likes to say, "there's more than one way to skin a cat."

Remember that.

So when people throw comments at you about the best way to conceive, the best way to birth, the best way to parent, the best way to worship, the best way to do anything – remember: Ashley talked about skinning a cat in her IVF book.

It will help the comparison-itis.

If you're going through infertility right now, then you know what I'm talking about. Usually, we like to overanalyze and worry about everything.

Ever heard of 'line eyes' or 'VVVFL'? Or even inverting a pregnancy test photo to see if the negative colors show a line? If you don't know what I'm talking about, stay tuned-you'll learn. If you do know what I'm talking about... I see you, I feel you, and we aren't alone.

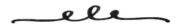

I read somewhere that one in seven couples experience infertility issues.

That statistic seemed high, and it didn't seem to affect any of the people attending our high school. Must have been the water. Some of our classmates started popping out babies at eighteen. Heck, Josh's brother and his wife had had three by the time they were in their early twenties. Josh himself was one of three children. His mother was one of nine. His father is one of four—a fertile-ass family. Josh's family was clearly shooting silver bullets. Though, to be fair, some of his mom's siblings were adopted, still: a fertile family. Plus, with me being a goody two shoes that never did anything wrong or off-schedule, I'd probably get pregnant the month we started trying.

How wrong I was.

Three

CHANDLER BING JUST RECEIVED the news that his sperm had low motility and I chuffed out a laugh at his response. It was twelve-thirty in the morning. I was in bed with the lights off, waiting for Josh to text me that he was on his way home.

His first job out of college was for a manufacturing engineering position on the second shift. He could work normal hours during his training period, which was only a couple of months. But once that was complete, he was officially moved to second shift. That meant that depending on what was happening with the machines on the floor, he might leave work at midnight or, on rougher nights, at four am. Depending on how I was feeling and if he was going to get home earlier, I would sometimes try to stay awake to see him. That's what I was planning to do tonight, hence the Friends marathon.

My phone lit up next to me on the bed. I peeked over and it was a text from Josh saying that he would be at least another hour. I sighed, put my phone on our headboard, and curled back down with my iPad.

I finished watching Chandler and Monica get their options from the doctor and shut off the screen. I stashed the tablet on my headboard next to my phone and tried to think happy thoughts. *Friends* was my favorite tv show, and the episodes rarely failed to make me smile. Chandler was hilarious with his sharp wit and quips, but my personality was eerily similar to Monica's. I had *Friends* T-shirts, trivia games, all the seasons on DVD, and even displayed some memorable quotes at our wedding. For example, I framed the quote 'he's her lobster' and displayed it at the reception. It was in a purple frame that matched the one in Monica's apartment, and I added cute, little red lobster images on either side of the quote. Before we left for the honeymoon, I had placed the frame on my dresser when we unpacked our wedding day bags. It hadn't moved in six months.

I nestled deeper into my pillow as I thought about how much life had changed since the wedding. Not only was Josh working second shift, which meant he headed into work at two in the afternoon and then came home in the wee hours of the morning, but it was also my first tax season in public accounting. So, on top of only being able to see my husband on weekends, I was also stressed to the max and felt like a complete failure.

I was unprepared for tax season's stress and hours. I had little training for my job (besides college classes) and was expected to sink or swim. Which really wasn't how I operated best. I received this job offer when I was in the first semester of my Master's degree in an Accounting program. Much like my classmates, I accepted the proposal by the time finals were over. Then, because I'm a planner by nature, I started my CPA exams during my spring semester. My plan was to be done with exams by the time I started working after graduation. Oh, and I was also planning our wedding. And after graduation, I was also fixing up the house we got on foreclosure. By the time I started my job, I had two of the four CPA exams complete, a foreclosed house we had mostly fixed up, and a wedding partially planned. Thankfully, by the time our wedding day arrived, the other two exams were passed and off my radar.

The CPA practice that I joined was not the most up-to-date. No paperless systems were in place, no working from home, nada. I was in the office all day, every day, including Saturdays. There were other firms out there that demanded more hours than mine did during tax season. But fresh out of college with no other benchmark? I was unprepared for the lifestyle change that tax season required.

And it was especially draining because I felt like I was doing *terribly*.

I didn't receive much training and had never completed a tax return. I felt like everything I touched was incorrect and that I couldn't do a single return correctly. It was mentally exhausting to feel like I was failing at my job day in, day out. During tax season, I was working Saturdays as well, so Sundays became precious to us.

I was nearing my breaking point.

We'd been stealing lunches together during the week just so we could see each other and catch up, but that wasn't enough. I missed my best friend. This wasn't what marriage was supposed to be like. This week had been rough as we slogged towards the April 15 deadline, and I just wanted to hug my husband. Or, as I was now calling him, 'my roommate.'

This wasn't a part of my plan. We were supposed to work, travel, do fun things, and pay down debt. Bucket list things! Then, we were going to have two-point-five kids, a golden retriever, a house with a white picket fence, and children's laughter always floating through our home. Not this endless silence in our house whenever I got home from work. Not this loneliness. Not this heartache.

I squeezed my eyes tighter and pulled a pillow towards me to cuddle. Tax season would be over soon. Josh's time on second shift would be over soon. It wouldn't be like this for long. Then our life could begin.

It won't be like this for long; I repeated this in my head, over and over, until I couldn't help the tears from seeping out of the corners of my eyes. I didn't bother wiping them away. I just pushed deeper into the pillow. I missed my best friend, and there wasn't much that I could do about it. I quietly cried until sleep claimed me.

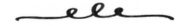

"Good morning, my little tax accountant!" Josh bellowed as he walked into our bedroom.

Maybe bellow was too strong a word, but in my sleepy state, it sure felt like one.

"Ugh," I groaned, pushing my head deeper into the pillows.

"Up and at 'em. I have a big day planned for us today. Lots of Jashley time." He had dubbed our celebrity couple name Jashley back in high school, and it just kind of stuck.

Josh had taken the day after April 15 off from work and spent the day with me (I already had it as a vacation day). I hoped that this day would recharge not only my battery but also lessen the downwards funk surrounding me.

"First order of business - brunch at the diner on Main. Then, I have a tee time booked at the club, then we can follow it up with some savory crepes, and we can end the day at home with pizza and a movie. During the said movie, you'll get a neck rub." He proudly outlined his events for the day.

None of that sounded bad, but he could have scheduled a nap somewhere in there.

"I have the truck loaded up with our clubs and shoes, and I already added water and snacks to the cooler. So get. Your ass. Up!"

"Alright, alright, alright," I grumbled as I rolled out of bed. I went to the closet and pulled out a polo and some pants that would be comfortable enough to golf in. I had an interesting body type that was the bane of my existence. I had good ol' child-bearing hips and a giant booty which made shopping for pants that could fit over my muscular thighs and big butt a real 'pain in the butt.' My arms were always strong from growing up around horses and playing sports. Throwing hay bales was the best softball workout that anyone could imagine. So my torso was strong as well, but my boobs were...there. I guess. I was constantly wearing ill-fitting bras because my ribcage was wide, but my chest was not. Buying a golf outfit as a whole? Frustrating. I'd have to find a medium polo and then try to see if they had a large, or sometimes extra large depending on the fit, for the pants, capris, or skirt. Don't even get me started on bathing suit sizing.

After finding golf clothes that could fit me after my signature 'winter weight,' I went to my jewelry cabinet, found jewelry that would match my shirt, and finished up my outfit by grabbing a visor.

Josh was waiting in the kitchen for me when I made my way downstairs. Finally, we headed out to the car and were on our way.

We were sitting in the diner, eating our pancakes, when my phone dinged from my pocket. I finished my bite of delicious Belgian waffle and took out my phone. Because in the order of priorities - breakfast foods always came first. My face unlocked the phone, and a message from my friend Megan previewed across the screen:

Scott and I talked last night, and we've started trying for a baby!!!!

I let out an "oh my God!" in excitement and texted her back. Josh looked up from his triple-decker stack of peanut butter, and chocolate chip pancakes smothered in strawberry syrup and grunted in question. His breakfast choices made me cringe.

"Megan just texted me. She said that she and Scott are going to try for a baby!" I was having a hard time containing my excitement in the crowded diner. Megan and I met years ago during my first internship and have stayed in touch since. We went to each other's weddings and texted almost daily. However, she had moved away a couple of years ago, so we didn't physically see each other anymore. So we were basically the world's best e-pen pals.

"She's been trying to convince Scott for a while, and he's been dragging his feet about getting on board because of his new job. I guess she wore him down!" My excitement was making me jittery.

Josh smiled at me, "another one bites the dust! Before you know it, all our friends will pop out babies!"

Hmm, that's a thought. I could be Team Baby...

"We did just pay off another one of the college loans last month, dear. We could join the ranks. We've thrown a ton of money at them this past year and have made a huge dent. Our monthly payments went from twelve hundred to seven hundred. It will be even less with my tax season bonus, and by the time nine months pass, we'll have even more chipped away. Plus, FMLA would protect us from parental leave by then because we would have surpassed our one-year mark. And we could start saving up on vacation time now! We could join the ranks!"

"You've given this a lot more thought than I have. I'm just not ready. And I don't think you can say that you are. You've been miserable the last few months. Are you planning on staying at this job? Are you going to be job searching soon? Are you willing to possibly be home with the baby solo while I'm at work? We talked the other day about how there might be a change in scheduling for my department, but nothing is set in stone yet. So, I very well might be on second shift until a new job opens up. I don't want that for you. I don't want that for me. And I wouldn't want that for our baby. To never see how his or her parents co-parent but just hand him or her off while the other heads out to work?"

"Yeah, you're right," I mumbled unconvincingly.

"I just don't think we're there yet. We have time. Let's get this work situation straightened out, and then we can talk more?" He asked.

"Yes, dear," I grumbled back. "I'm still happy for Megan, though. She's been trying to get him on board since our wedding. So it took him a bit to come around. I'm glad she convinced him."

"Is he still doing recruiting for that college baseball team?"

And, just like that, over good conversation, delicious breakfast foods, and apple juice, I forgot about how miserable I had been the last few months and just soaked up the time with my husband. But the second my fella said 'go,' we were going to start trying because *I was more than ready to experience the joys of being a mom.*

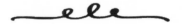

I threw a hard right jab with determination but zero talent. I chased it with a left cross that felt equally uncoordinated—then finished with a right uppercut.

I had reconnected with one of my friends from high school in the last couple of months since tax season ended. She talked me into doing kickboxing classes with her. In one of my weaker moments, I bought a 25-session card. I was in my eleventh class but saw no noticeable improvement in my technique. It was probably time to concede - maybe kickboxing wasn't for me.

We finished the class covered in sweat, smiling, and tired. I found that being physical kept my mind exhausted enough that I didn't focus on the fact that I missed my husband like crazy.

"See you on Thursday!" I called out as I headed to my car. I loaded up my small bag with my gloves and indoor sneakers and took out my duffel bag from the back seat. I threw on some softball cleats, changed tops, and drove over to our local ball fields for our under-the-lights game.

Kickboxing tired me out physically, but softball served an entirely different purpose. It gave me a social outlet that I hadn't had in years. I had eleven other girls on the team (and their significant others and children) to socialize with to fill that void of friendship that was missing since coming back from college. Twice a week, we got together and battled one of the five other teams in the league for nothing more than bragging rights.

Most of the teams consisted of pretty relaxed players who were just there to have a good time. However, there was one team that every league must have that took everything entirely too seriously. Luckily, that was not who we played that night. Too much drama came from playing that team. It took away some of the fun.

I got to the field relatively early and had time to stretch, play catch, and socialize before our game.

"Hey there, Karli!" I called to a toddler who was wearing a mini version of our team uniform.

"Ball! Ball! Ball!" She held a softball in her hands and unevenly made her way toward me.

"She just learned how to really whip that thing, so watch out," her dad, Mark, said as he came up behind her.

"She's going to play catcher, just like her mom!" My friend and teammate Lisa proudly declared. Karli was a good blend of both of her parents. She got her mom's beautiful caramel skin and her dad's stunning blue eyes. It was a wonderful combination. Then add in her toothy grin and rosy cheeks, and you would think you were looking at a real-life American Girl doll.

I hoped my future children would be as adorable as she was because Lordy, she was precious.

"I thought we agreed she was going to run track?" Mark chimed in from his kneeling position near Karli. She was trying to throw the ball at his head, and he was dodging, retrieving, and handing back to her. She thought it was hilarious and was laughing maniacally.

"Well, whatever she does, it's fine by me," Lisa amended.

Mark and Lisa met in college and took some time to set up their careers before jumping into the parenthood pool. They were a couple of years older than Josh and me, but we had very similar interests and personalities, so they were the couple that I gravitated to most when I joined the team. On random Sundays, we'd go to their house to watch whatever soccer game was on TV. Josh and Mark would talk shop about the Champion's League while Lisa and I would chat about Karli and life. Whenever Josh and I visited them and played with Karli, she would wrap us a little tighter around her finger. The child was adorable, and I'd grown super attached to the little munchkin.

I bent down closer to her, "Hey there, cutie!" Then, I put my hands out invitingly, "can you throw me the ball?" And just like that, I was promptly rewarded for my efforts with a ball chucked at me.

I did a little jump out of the way, gave big eyes to her dad behind her, and went to retrieve the ball. He gave me a look that said, 'better you than me–I've been stuck doing this for the last thirty minutes.' Maybe she wouldn't play any sports. Maybe she'd train dogs because she had this fetch thing down.

"So, when are you and Josh going to have kids?" Lisa asked.

"Oh my God, I know," I stressed. "I'm so ready. But we're just trying to pay off some debt first so we can set ourselves and kids up for the best possible life." I repeated our refrain of the last almost year.

"You have time. Enjoy the freedom while you have it." Mark reassured me.

"Don't wait too long, or our kids won't grow up together!" Lisa contradicted.

"Yes, I'm sure she's going to base her procreation decision on our kids' ages." Mark countered back.

Lisa sniffed prissily and rolled the ball at her feet back to Karli. Karli promptly threw the ball behind herself by accident.

"We have time, but sooner rather than later would be my preference," I added softly, watching Karli figure out where the ball went.

"Just don't wait too long," Lisa added. "Once you hit like thirty-four, the risk of complications doubles or something like that. And if you guys want more than two kids..." Karli had turned around and realized she had rolled the ball behind her and waddled over to it.

"Yeah, I know." I agreed distractedly. "I know." Karli picked up the ball and held it out proudly towards me as if to say, 'I found it! Aren't I incredible!'

"Ball!" she squealed happily.

As we played with Karli and waited for the game before us to end, a couple of other family members of teammates wandered over from where they were hanging out on the playground. The team was mostly made up of women that were about five years older than me. And mostly, they were on the stage where they had kids that would come to the games. There were a couple of outliers on our team, as any women's softball team has. One player was in her forties, and one was in her teens. Without having Josh there as my wingman, I got to know the players, spouses, and their kids very well, or else I would have been awkwardly sitting on the bench or by the fence all summer long. A few kids formed a rough and tumble friendship, and they would run about the playground next to the softball field the entire night. You could hear them laughing and yelling from the field. One memorable moment was when an older brother tried to prevent his younger brother from playing with them, and they were fighting by the swings. Our shortstop yelled at them from her position on the field and laid down the hammer. They were ordered to either let everyone play, or that they wouldn't come back. It quieted the protests, and though we heard grumbling and whining, we didn't hear any more fighting.

I wondered how Josh and I would parent.

One teammate, Brittany, had a six-month-old, and whenever she ran from base to base, she'd hold her boobs to her chest and talk about it being "liquid gold." The other moms would chuckle and get into the joys, or not-so joys, of breastfeeding. As a bottle-fed baby myself, I learned a lot from those conversations. Maybe more than I ever really wanted to know about birth, babies, and breastfeeding, but I couldn't deny that it was certainly educational. *I could be ready for this.*

I learned that several of my teammates had suffered miscarriages in the past. It was much more common than I thought. I learned nipple cream is a must when it comes to breastfeeding and that milk blisters were terrible. I learned you could pee when running from first to second, second to third, from third to home, or generally anytime when you sneeze after you've given birth. And that your vagina is never the same. One of the weirder things I heard from the husbands is that they hated the postpartum times when they'd have to clean out clumps of hair from their shower drains from their wives' shedding.

So, all in all, even though I enjoyed playing softball and keeping busy, it gave me an emotional outlet that I had been missing. But it also brought to the forefront of my mind every time I saw my team that I was meant to be a mom, and I wasn't yet. I knew I "had time," as everyone liked to remind me. But I was ready. I wanted a baby of my own—time to revisit that conversation with the hubs.

Four

"I GOT THE PROMOTION!" Josh exclaimed in my ear as I was pushing my golf cart to my ball on the ninth hole.

"No way! That's awesome! When do you get to move to normal hours?" I shot thumbs up to my mom and dad as I pulled out my pitching wedge and waved them onto their balls. I felt a weight lift from my shoulders with his words.

"They said I can jump back to regular first shift hours starting next week. They're getting rid of all second-shift engineering support ASAP, so I'll be able to be human again! Wait, I'm being paged on the radio. Gotta go. Love you. Bye,"

I heard a quick click after I said my goodbyes and smiled hugely at my parents, who were waiting for me to hit.

"Josh is going to move to the first shift next week!"

"Oh, Ash, that's awesome!" My mom echoed my feelings from earlier.

"So next week, I'll be paying for an additional cart when we play?" My dad asked dryly. "But really, I'm happy for him, and he deserves it."

Josh put in for a change of shift at work a couple of weeks ago. He was waiting to hear the news. His company was at the tail end of deciding what they wanted to do about their off-shift support. But it sounded like they decided to can the idea altogether. I was getting my husband back.

Tax season had been over for a little over a month, and Josh and I had taken up golfing on our weekends together. During the week, I now had softball and golf. I chose not to renew my kickboxing card. I was getting pretty good at golf. I think it translated well from my field hockey and softball experiences. Josh wasn't as natural at it, but he was athletic enough to make up for the difference. We both had some impressive slices, but given that he was a lefty, our slices put us on opposite sides of the fairways. We constantly tried to continue our conversations with each other long after leaving the realm of earshot, and we'd have to tell the offending speaker, "You're gonna to have a bad time!" The subtext being, 'you're going to have a bad time continuing to talk if you think I can hear you because you're just going to repeat yourself.' We started to use that around the house as well. If someone was talking while the other was in the shower... "you're gonna have a bad time!" If someone was talking while the other was walking into the basement... "you're gonna have a bad time!" It was somewhat of a catchphrase of ours now.

With Josh going to the first shift, we'd have more opportunities to repeat it to each other! I could feel my spirits lift the more I thought about it. We could finally be newlyweds. My heart was singing!

We finished up our round of golf and were sitting in the clubhouse when some friends of my dad came by our table.

"Bobby. Mary." The shortest of the bunch said as he walked towards my dad. He did the type of handshake that held the right hand trapped in a handhold and the left hand clasping the other person's shoulder. His white hair puffed out around the bottom of his golf hat, and he had a white shirt with red lobsters all over it, along with red matching shorts. He was adorable.

My dad greeted him happily. "Hey there, old-timer. How are ya? You remember my daughter, Ashley?" My dad gestured over to me with a wave of his hand once it was freed.

"Yes, yes. The golf prodigy that wasn't. Your father told me about your newfound passion for golf. He said you'll be kicking his butt in no time!" My father was a nine-handicap. I was a max. No kicking of his butt would ever occur in this lifetime.

"That would be something to see!" I agreed. "If I ever get that good, I'll need to buy a lottery ticket that night to capitalize on whatever else Lady Luck left with me!"

"Gah!" He chuckled good-naturedly, and he waved his friends to go on to their tables without him. "Where's your husband tonight? Didn't want to golf in the rain showers?"

"No, no, he's still at work. Though he received good news today that he'd be able to work normal hours again soon."

"He's in charge of second shift engineering support over at his facility, so he works from two to midnight or so." My dad added in for context.

"Well, that's hard! How are you supposed to get on giving your parents some grandkids if you two are working opposite shifts? Being a grandfather is the best thing that's ever happened to me. You think you love your kids. But then when that grandkid arrives? Game over. I have two grandbabies right now. Both girls. They love their grandpa, that's for sure. They know that when Grandpa is around, they get to do a lot of things that their mom and dad don't allow." He smiled conspiratorially at my parents. "Hype them up on sugar and movies and send them home." He lowered his voice as if in secret. "You can get all the same loves and memories as when your own kids were young, except you get to send them home when it's bedtime or when they're cranky." He paused again and looked back at me. "You've been married for a while now. Time to get on that!"

I smiled back at him (though, truth be told, I was uncomfortable talking about making babies with an almost stranger. Heck, I was uncomfortable even *thinking* about talking about making babies with my family. Nope, no discussions would be had about that).

"We're working on paying down some debt first," I deflected.

But now that Josh would be working a normal shift...

"Nonsense! Debt will always be there! There's never a right time for having kids. You just have them, and everything moves around them to make it work."

"Ahh, okay. I'll let Josh know," I said jokingly.

He chuckled and patted my dad on the back. "She gets her humor from you! Alright, great seeing you guys. I'm off to collect my winnings from today's round from the boys. It pays to hit from the whites." He winked at me and walked through the winding tables to where his party was sitting and chatting. He stopped three times to clasp people on the shoulders, rib them good-naturedly, or say hello.

"He's such a nice guy," my mom chimed in, now that he had left earshot.

"He is. He's doing a project for us at work this summer. It's been a bit of a bear—just one thing after another keeps going wrong. But he's just rolling with the punches and just figures out the next thing to do. He's been great to work with and to keep the crews moving." My dad and uncles owned several businesses in the area and had fingers in many pies. My boss, Bill, was the CPA for all the accounts. Because of independence requirements, I wasn't associated with any of that work, but I was about 85% sure my family ties were why I got my job with Bill in the first place. Who wants to *not* hire the relative of a big client? Talk about awkward. Poor Bill. I hope I didn't make him regret his decision to take me on because the one thing that would be more awkward than not hiring the relative of important clients would be firing her.

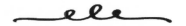

"Fore!"

My stomach pitched, and I quickly threw my arms up over my head and bent my knees awkwardly. After a second, I looked up and glared daggers at my darling husband from across the fairway.

"Sorry!" He called out sheepishly.

I held his look for half a second more and then bent down to pick up my club. We just had the conversation two minutes ago that I would hit first and then get out of his line of fire, as his balls had developed a tendency to follow me around the fairway. My best guess what that he got impatient and was overconfident in his ability to control his shot.

It had been two months since his schedule switched from second shift to first. Life was everything I had hoped it would be. Unless he had soccer or I had softball, we would meet after work at our favorite golf course and play until the sun went down. Our family membership gave us unlimited golfing for the rest of the year. We were taking advantage of every penny spent. Both of us had gotten better, but that wasn't saying much. Going from losing ten balls per round to losing two wasn't enough to get us on the PGA tour, but we were proud of ourselves, and that's all that mattered.

"Sorry, dear," Josh repeated to me as he came up behind where my ball was lying.

"I can't believe you'd put the baby and me in jeopardy like that!"

"Ha! Like you'd be able to keep a secret that long to announce it to me on a golf course. Though that would be a heck of a way to tell me. Do that. Tell me about it on a golf course when you finally get pregnant. Or before I go to a soccer game. Something big. Because that would totally amp me up."

"I'll do my best." I chuckled as we started walking toward our next shots. They landed close to each other, so it was a walk where we didn't need to bookmark our conversation before branching off towards our own balls.

"Wait, you're not pregnant, are you?"

"No, dear. I was just kidding." I assured him dryly, my eyebrows furrowed.

"Okay, good."

I looked at him quickly to see him adding his shot metrics onto his phone. We took the plunge a month ago and agreed we could start "softly" trying. What Josh called "not trying but not preventing either." I stopped taking *The Pill* when we got engaged because I read that it can take the reproductive system a while to get back on track after being on it for a while. So really, the only change had been the absence of condoms. His comment made me suspicious of how 'on board' he really was. What does 'okay good' mean?

"These past few months have just been brutal," I said to him.

"More headaches and cramps?" He paused slightly, "and mood swings?" He tacked on the last as if it were an afterthought.

"Headache, cramps, spotting, insatiable hunger, acne. I'm over it. Just knock me up already." It was like my body knew I was trying to get pregnant and gave me a taste of the misery coming my way. I felt like I was fifteen and going through the intense parts of puberty all over again.

He threw back his head and laughed. "From what you've told me each night, those things definitely don't sound like they go away with pregnancy!"

He wasn't wrong. I had jumped in headfirst into the TTC world. First lesson: no one calls it 'trying to conceive.' Everyone on the apps and boards calls it by the shorthand 'TTC.' There were acronyms for everything. AF stood for Aunt Flow, aka your period. BD stood for baby dance, aka sex. There was talk of baby dust, DS#1 (dear son number 1), BFNs and BFPs (big fat no's and big fat positives), and VVVFL (very very very faint lines seen on pregnancy tests). I learned that red dye tests were more reliable than blue dye tests, and I relearned about the birds and the bees. High school health class did *not* prepare me for this. Of course, I shared these reproductive information nuggets with Josh, and he would remind me we weren't really "trying trying" yet. Just again, "not preventing." To which I'd assure him I knew, he'd roll his eyes, and then I kept researching.

"Well. No." I dragged out. "I know they don't go away. But at least there's a reason for it. A light at the end of the tunnel, so to speak." I rolled my eyes.

"That light ends up being a freight train out of your vagina."

I scowled. He smiled cheekily back.

"You're probably feeling gross because of the stress of tax season. So that's normal. Also, the doc said it could take a while to get pregnant after being on the pill for so long. So don't be getting impatient."

It's not like I stopped taking it a month ago - it had been about two years since I came off it. I felt justified in my impatience.

"I'm not." I lied.

"Liar," he shot back.

I grinned back at him and kept walking toward my ball.

"You're lucky I love you and can't say no to you," he called good-naturedly.

He wasn't wrong. He spoiled me, and even if he weren't 100% sure he wanted to try for a baby, if he felt that strong against it, we'd stop in a heartbeat and pump the brakes. So I knew he was just getting off on giving me a hard time.

"I know, dear. I love you too."

"There's no one else I'd rather give shit to," he called out.

I smiled up at him from lining up my shot. "Same."

I pulled back my club. I was perfectly balanced. This shot was going to be perfect. I could feel it. A fraction of a second away from my club hitting the ball, an excessive coughing fit erupted from my husband. My ball shanked to the left and into the woods. I looked up at him slowly in disbelief and saw him grinning at me. "You were winning by a stroke," he explained as he held up his phone. He shrugged and walked towards his own ball. My laughter damn near shook the trees.

He'd be an awesome dad.

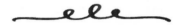

The summer and fall passed in a blur. It was the most amazing time of my life. We'd meet almost every day after work and just go golfing until the sun set. Or go to my softball game. Or to one of his soccer or Rugby games. We soaked up our time together, making up for the lost time. But before we knew it, winter came, and it was tax season again. This was my second tax season, and it was going much better than the first... *loads better.* Worlds better! But I was having what Josh was starting to call 'a moment.' At this point, even with the experience, I couldn't get this damn trial balance actually to balance. Balance was *in the name!* How hard could it be?

I had checked the columns twice and wasn't finding the difference, and it was driving me bonkers.

A shadow passed my office door, and a man in a winter coat was walked out of the building by my boss, Bill.

I hadn't recognized him, but there had been an influx of unfamiliar faces meeting with Bill over the last couple of weeks, so I just figured I'd be learning who they were soon enough when their tax documents came in for me to prep.

I sighed as I looked back at my screen. I lost where I was—time to start again.

I changed my music station to something with classical music, so I didn't run into oncoming traffic. I went and refilled my water bottle and sat back down. But before I could jump back into the 'Trial Balance That Wasn't,' my phone vibrated softly on my desk.

I looked over to it and saw a text from my mom asking Josh and me over for dinner Thursday night–she was making Fettucine Alfredo, my favorite. I shot her back a quick affirmative and then sent one to Josh, letting him know we were going there for dinner.

As I relocked my phone, I sighed again. I briefly reflected on the past few months. I had to admit that everything was a bit weird. Work was going great, and I was officially a CPA. I was doing much better than I had last year. Tax prep was coming along much easier, and I was developing a nice rapport with my clients. *This* was what I wanted out of my career. And it was glorious seeing Josh every day. But I was getting antsy about the lack of progress in the conception game. I should have been pregnant by now. We had been having unprotected sex for about *ten months*. I'd been tracking my cycles and jumping Josh's bones (or should I say bone) whenever it was around 'that time.' I think he was getting exhausted! But still nothing.

My cycles had never been regular, so it was hard to tell exactly what was considered 'late' or when I'd be ovulating. I could range from a 21-day cycle to a 34-day cycle. The window left something to be desired.

But I was trying to handle it the best I could. I wasn't a person who could just go with the flow. I was a planner. I liked the order. There were pro-con lists for everything. I had an excel household budget that was updated monthly. We had amortization tables for our student and vehicle loans. I was a person who thrived with order and structure. When the unplanned happened, or in this case, didn't happen, it caused me to fixate and stress.

So now, rather than just stressing about this stupid trial balance, I was also worried about what could be wrong as to why we weren't getting pregnant. *Great.*

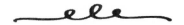

I ran through all the numbers again and, an hour later, found that there was a combination of a negative number where it should have been a positive and a transposition error. Eureka! I hit save before a meteor could hit our power grid, making me lose the work I just put in.

"Hi Ashley, can I show you something?" Bill asked as he came into my office.

"Sure," I said as I stood up to stand next to him. It made me uncomfortable to stay seated while people talked to me. It felt much more comfortable to stand when they were standing. He had a tax return page in his hand with some red pencil scratched on it. He held it in front of us and explained what I did wrong and the better way to do that type of reporting. His hand was shaking as he held the page, making it hard to see what he wrote in his chicken scratch. I peered up at him.

"Do you want a candy? Is your sugar low?"

"What? No, no, I'm fine. My wife would kill me if I ate candy. I'll have lunch when I'm done reviewing this one. I just wanted to explain this while I was thinking of it."

"Okay, just let me know." I reiterated. He didn't look sick, but his hand was still trembling. As he walked out, I made a mental note to swing by his office in a few minutes to ensure I caught him eating something. I sat back down and jumped into chipping away at my seemingly endless tax return prep queue.

Five

A COUPLE OF WEEKS later, I walked into work with a gym bag over one shoulder, my purse on the other, and a smile for our receptionist. The boss man shot a hello back after I called out a quick hi. I walked down the hall to my office. Quipping a quick hello to his wife, whose office was across from me, and their son, who was also a CPA at the firm and had the office on the other side of mine. Working for a firm run by a family was usually cool; it only ever got awkward when there was a disagreement between family members. But for the most part, it was the exact environment I craved - very family-friendly. Despite the lack of on-the-job training and the stress of tax season, that is.

The firm's owner, Bill, was a total sap for his grandkids. His son, Mike, had two little kids who would come in to visit him during the day and would always swing by my office to say hi. They loved me. I'm sure it had nothing to do with the candy I gave them. Visiting with them would always prompt me to fantasize about what it would be like when my kids were big enough to come to visit Mommy at work. I couldn't wait!

It was three o'clock, and I worked through lunch again. I usually hit up the gym next door every day during lunch, but I was deep into a complicated tax return and didn't want to lose my momentum. The entire office was a little tense because of the upcoming March 15 tax deadline, but so far, it was going much better than the year before. My total breakdowns for this tax season numbered at zero. Which was incredible given how many

I had the year before. Actually, this tax season was downright pleasant. I finally caught my rhythm in public accounting. I came in around seven thirty in the morning, worked until lunch, then I would walk to the gym and work out for an hour. After that, I returned to the office and worked until dinner. I'd then go home, cuddle up with Josh, and talk about our days. It was what I pictured life would be like when I first accepted the job, and I was relieved that it was finally coming to fruition.

I had been hitting the gym pretty hard at lunchtime for two main reasons: first, I wanted to be as healthy as possible when I got pregnant (which still hadn't happened yet, and I was stressing), and second because it was a great stress relief.

We had moved from the 'not preventing' to the 'actively trying' stage back in September when we hit our first wedding anniversary. We had sent a whopper of a check to the student loan company that had decimated our savings, but it paid off several of our smaller loans. There were still plenty left. But, with the decreased monthly payment, we agreed we could start getting serious. During a Black Friday sale in November, we got a wild hair and bought a crib for our spare bedroom. In December, during one of the Christmas sales, we saw a recliner for sale that looked like heaven, and we added that to our new nursery. With each passing month, I got a little more restless. Josh was still unflappable and calm about everything. It helped calm me a little, but I was a completely healthy twenty-six-year-old. There was no reason that I could see preventing me from being pregnant by now.

We had been 'not preventing' for a few months shy of a year and actively trying for a little less than that. So, like my typical self, I dove into the message boards and TTC apps. The information I gleaned from them didn't ease my fears at all. Instead, it's almost like an internal clock had started in my mind. I couldn't wait for the summer when I could go into my doctor's office and say that we'd been having unprotected sex for a year, time for them to help us pinpoint why we weren't getting anywhere. Because, apparently, doctors wouldn't see someone in my age range until they had been trying for at least a year. But in the meantime, I went online and ordered a bunch of Ovulation Predictor Kits (OPKs). There was a boxed option that allowed you to buy the OPKs and HPTs (Home Pregnancy Tests) in bulk. They weren't anything fancy, just tiny test strips, but with the frequency with which I was burning through them, I needed to be efficient with my TTC funds because my insurance didn't cover those puppies.

I finished my accounting journal entry in the software and looked up as my boss came to my office door. "Do you have a minute? Mike and I want to talk to you."

"Sure. Do you need me to bring my status list?" I tried to find where my notes were on the status of my tax returns but stopped when he replied.

"No, this is something different." He was wringing his hands and seemed a little nervous. "I'll meet you in the conference room."

I got up and followed him into the small conference room that we only ever used for team meetings and client conferences. Mike was already sitting in a chair by the door, so I took the chair opposite him, and then Bill sat at the head of the table immediately to my left.

"So, I'm guessing you've already heard the news..."

My stomach plummeted. He had been acting weird for the last month. He was constantly out of the office, which I thought was for client meetings. But weeks ago, he was holding that piece of paper while talking to me about a return, and his hand was shaking like a leaf. I thought it was strange, but I assumed his sugar was low.

Oh my God. He was sick. He was going to tell me he had cancer.

My heart started racing. My clothes immediately felt too heavy and hot.

I looked over at his son sitting across from me. He was watching me silently.

"No," I replied. "What happened? Are you okay?"

"Your dad hasn't said anything to you?" Bill seemed surprised.

My parents had been clients of Bill's for as long as I could remember. In fact, my grandparents were his clients when he first started out on his own. So my family had known him forever. I was 99% sure that's the only reason I got the job offer. However, I hope I kept it based on my merit–not my family's business relationships.

"No," I repeated, but now more curious than concerned. My foot started bouncing under the table, and I started using my pointer finger to scratch at my thumb cuticle to channel my nerves. My eyes scanned his face, wondering what I was seeing. He didn't look sick exactly, just nervous and tired.

"Well, Mike has taken some time to reevaluate his life and his work-life balance in public accounting," He began. My eyes shot to Mike, who sat there quietly, "And he's decided to make the change to private accounting."

"Okay." I dragged out. This didn't sound terrible. My pulse slowed.

"And, as you may remember, when I hired you, we talked about how Mike would eventually run this firm as my succession plan. The hope was to train you up and give you enough experience and knowledge that you two could build it into whatever you wanted it to be."

Again, I nodded. I remembered the plan. I based most of my life expectations for the last year and a half on this plan.

"Well, because Mike has decided to switch out of public and I've been looking towards retiring, that only left me with a couple of options... Your dad really didn't talk to you?" He confirmed again.

I was starting to get nervous again. "No, he hasn't said anything to me," I assured him.

"Oh. Well, anyway... I decided I needed to do what was best for my clients. Most have been with me for forty-five years. So I wanted to ensure they weren't just left high and dry. I've been talking with other firms about buying my book of business." Again, he paused and looked at me quizzically.

What was I missing? Why were both of them looking at me like that?

"And I've found a firm that I think will be a great fit for my clients and be able to offer them an exceptional level of service. They have staff that is up to date on all the different audit rules and tax code workings and are much more experienced and knowledgeable on many topics. In addition, they have dedicated subject experts, where I've always considered myself more of a generalist."

I nodded mutely, still waiting for the other shoe to drop.

"We've reached an agreement, and they'll be buying the firm. They'll start taking over clients this summer, and Mike and I will help transition some of the larger accounts and make sure that the transition goes as smooth as possible."

I felt like an idiot, but I nodded again and shot a look over to Mike. He was looking at me expectantly, but also... sadly?

"What I'm trying to say is, I don't think they'll be keeping you. They are probably going to staff everything here with employees they already have. Right down to reception, so we'll talk to Janet in a few minutes too. But we wanted to let you know and to tell you that we're more than happy to give you a recommendation wherever, but you should probably start looking soon. I'll keep you on the payroll as long as I need to, but... you should start looking." He said this last part quickly, like ripping off a Band-Aid.

My heart stopped. Oh my God. Realization hit.

I was being fired, or more technically, laid off. But still. I was losing my job. My career. My plan!

I looked back and forth between Mike and Bill rapidly. My fingers stopped fidgeting. My foot stopped tapping.

My vision narrowed.

Oh my God. What if I was pregnant? I'd have to job hunt for a position that would be okay with me taking time off after the baby was born, even though I wouldn't have been there for a year.

What if I wasn't pregnant? I'd have to find a new job, and the responsible thing would be to work there for at least a year before taking time off to have a baby.

I went into public accounting, recognizing that I should time my procreation goals around tax season.

A new job and a restart on my longevity there would push everything back even more...

"Umm, okay." I began slowly. "Uh, that's good news that you're going to retire as you wanted." I squeezed out. The tears were building in the back of my throat. I looked at Mike. "And that's good that you've found something that will give you more time with the kids. Where are you going?"

"I don't have any plans yet. I'm going to take some time off, and then I'll decide."

He didn't even have a job lined up? That was a big life decision, and he didn't have something in the works?

Part of me was angry at him for being the catalyst that caused this upheaval in my life. I was *not* the type of person that handled change well!

Part of me understood and applauded him for making that leap. On the other hand, it couldn't have been easy to tell your dad that you didn't want any part of the company he built, which was his legacy.

But he had it made! He had the keys to the castle! He could have scheduled work so he wouldn't have had as many hours if he felt like he was missing out on his kids' lives. As the boss, he could have done whatever he wanted!

I ping-ponged back and forth on my emotions.

A thought struck me.

"You already told my dad?"

"Yes. We visited all the big business accounts yesterday and introduced them to the new shareholders."

He didn't tell me.

My dad didn't tell me I was about to lose my job.

I wanted to sob. That hurt worse than anything so far. My throat burned as I fought back the tears,

Instead, I kept a lid on it and tried to ask the polite questions: Timing, retirement plans, "you must be excited," "how does the wife feel," etc. But my heart wasn't in it.

Bill and Mike wrapped things up with me fairly quickly, and I robotically walked back to my office. I sat down and looked at the clock-half past three.

It seemed like a good day to leave early.

I shut off my computer and saw our receptionist enter the conference room.

I grabbed my unused gym bag, purse, and jacket and left the office, heading straight to my car. Of course, they'd probably wonder where I'd gone, but my guess was that they wouldn't wonder for long, given what they shared.

I called Josh when I got in the car.

"I just got fired." I choked out and then cried. "I need you to come home."

"What!" He asked, "What do you mean, you 'got fired.'"

I garbled something out, and he just said, "Never mind, I'll leave now and meet you at home."

Knowing that he had a forty-minute drive home just made me cry harder.

I got home before Josh and jumped in the shower. The water carried my tears away as I silently cried in the shower. I was probably being dramatic. People get laid off all the time. But again, I don't handle change well. Deviation from plans always caused me an excessive amount of stress. There might be a little undiagnosed anxiety and OCD in my personality, but as I usually had things under control, it never really impacted my life negatively.

When Josh got home, I explained what happened, and, like usual, he cut right to the point.

"So basically, you weren't fired. They just sold the business, and the new firm doesn't want to hire any new staff. You can stay on for however long it takes to find a new job. And they're willing to give you a great recommendation."

I sniffed wetly and then, feeling it was 'too wet,' blew my nose... Again.

"Correct."

"Okay then. This sucks, but it's not that big of a deal, Ash. We'll be okay,"

"My dad knew and didn't warn me!" I wailed.

"Did Bill tell you later that he asked your dad not to tell you?"

"Yeah. So?"

"So, it sounds like your dad respected your boss's wishes to tell you personally."

"Don't be reasonable right now! Be upset with me!"

"You're upset enough for both of us. I don't need to join in." He said in, I'm sure, what he thought was a soothing manner. Instead, it just got my hackles up.

"I'm going to ask him,"

"You're what? Ask who what?"

"I'm driving to my parents. Are you coming?"

"No, Ash. Don't do that. It serves no purpose."

"Okay, so you're staying here."

"Ash,"

I grabbed my keys and started walking out the door. When I got to the car, Josh nabbed my keys and told me to get in the passenger seat and that I shouldn't be driving. When we got to my parent's house, which was about five minutes down the road, I stormed in.

"You knew Bill was selling the firm and that I was losing my job, and you didn't *warn me*?" My voice broke on the last words, and the tears poured again.

The welcoming smile froze on my dad's face, and he just looked at me. Josh started rubbing my lower back softly.

"You knew and didn't tell me!" I choked out again.

"Ash. He asked me not to tell you. That he wanted to do it himself." He looked genuinely apologetic, but I couldn't help myself.

"But you're my dad! You knew! You should have told me. You could have warned me. You knew and should have warned me that I was losing my job. *You're my dad*" I started sobbing harder.

I often look back on this conversation and feel bad for my dad. He must have felt awful. Here I was, having a mental breakdown, and he was just doing what he thought was right.

The stress of having this curveball thrown at me during the height of tax season, during a few months of my life that I was already starting to question and worry about our fertility, was apparently enough to send me into hysterics. I cried some more at my parents' house, let Josh bring me home, and continued sobbing there. By the time bedtime came around, I was all cried out and had reached the acceptance stage. I was concerned that no other public accounting firm would be interested if I applied to them during or at the end of tax season. I worried that the stigma of job hunting so close to the end of tax season would imply that I was a poor performer and that maybe I was fired from my previous public accounting job. But hopefully, their willing recommendations would disprove that. I'd have to deal with that later. I just needed to get through the next month and a half, and then I could tackle the job market. But in the meantime, we'd have to put the TTC mission on hold. Finally, I found the silver lining and began my usual calculative planning. Meanwhile, my heart sank at the thought of waiting even longer to become pregnant.

Six

I SPENT THE NEXT month job searching while finishing up the rest of tax season. Josh and I had tabled the full-court press on TTC and decided to let the dust settle on things for a bit. Plus, we rationalized that if we got pregnant in April or May, I'd have a baby at the beginning of the next tax season, and that wouldn't be a good way to start my new tax season at a new firm. So we were back to not preventing but also not trying.

A week after tax season ended, I found a job posting online for a local CPA firm and applied immediately. The interview went well, and they asked me why I was looking for another public accounting job so soon after tax season ended. My guess was that they were afraid to hire someone who failed at another CPA firm and was subsequently laid off. They wouldn't want that person to come to them. But Bill was super clear I could inform prospective employers of my circumstance and that he would talk to them if they had any concerns. Sure enough, the prospective CPA firm managers called Bill and talked about me, and they felt comfortable offering me a job.

The job was almost the same as it was at Bill's firm, but they were much more technologically savvy. I was thrown into the world of a paperless office, which was incredible. I loved the paperless mentality. I was given an at-home setup and an office at their location, and they allowed me to work from home whenever I needed to. The commute was only ten minutes away from our house, and I enjoyed the switch. Despite the fear of the unknown, the devil you know vs. the devil you don't, I felt a lot more understood at the new firm. They had senior accountants that helped onboard me and filled in the gaps in my education and experience to make me an all-around better employee. They matched my previous salary, had a retirement plan, and offered pretty good health insurance, not that I needed it, I was usually very healthy. I think the only time I had been to the doctor's office in the last three years was to get off the pill, and then another visit when I broke my thumb catching during a softball game the previous summer.

The whole experience was a mini-life lesson for me; I felt ridiculous for panicking so thoroughly when Bill laid me off. I was (and still am) a planner, so I got a little freaked when life threw a curveball. But the job offer coming so quickly on the heels of my interview was an excellent reminder to stay positive and look for opportunities instead of focusing on the negatives. I'd need to remind myself of that lesson many more times during the upcoming trials.

After a few months on the job, I was approached about taking a job coaching field hockey at the local middle school. I asked my new employer if they would support that, and they were totally on board, so rather than golfing every day after work in the fall, I headed over to the middle school and got to coach a bunch of sixth, seventh, and eighth graders.

And. It. Was. Awesome.

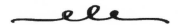

"Kiddo, for the love of God, be aware of who's around you when you're swinging your stick!"

I rushed over to the girl who had just taken a wayward swing directly to her face. The girl was bent over, crying, and grabbing her face. I squatted down quickly and pulled out my phone in case I had to call for help. I peeked up at her face.

Her hands covered most of it, but I could see where the stick had clipped her. Luckily, it looked like the eye protection took most of the impact and maybe slid off and onto her forehead a bit. It didn't look terrible, but it was certainly noticeable.

"Honey, are you okay? On a scale from one to ten, where are you with the pain?" I looked up at one of the other girls and nodded my head towards the athletic trainer, who was working on wrapping a hamstring injury for a soccer player. The girl darted off to bring her over.

"I'm, fuh-, fuh-, fine," she stuttered, pulling off her goggles. I pushed her into a seat. Our coaching first aid classes were great, but at the moment, I wasn't thinking out the steps as I should.

"We're getting the trainer over here, and she'll look at you. Then, she'll let us know what we need to do."

"No!" she burst out. "I don't want the trainer. I'm fine. Just give me a minute."

"Kiddo, I appreciate the commitment, but I'd never be able to live with myself if something was wrong. So just let her check you out really quick, and if everything's fine, then no big deal, you can keep playing."

"But if she says I'm hurt, I can't play in our game tomorrow!"

"Kiddo," I said placatingly. "Let's have her check you out and go from there."

The kids had come a long way. The season started with me making every rookie coaching mistake a person can make. There were the girls who were natural athletes, and then there were girls that could hardly walk a straight line. Some girls wanted to impress the coach and were 'eager to please.' Then some girls viewed the sport as a social avenue and didn't understand that running was a part of the sport. After ranting to my dad one night at a dinner at their house, he laid some truth bombs on me he had accumulated through his years of coaching softball.

"Each kid is different. For me, I always preferred coaching girls over boys. When I coached teams that your brother was on, I was just met with boy after boy who thought they knew it all. When I coached your teams, the girls I coached were much more willing to learn and try new things. But either way, each kid has their own home life, skillset, and personality.

It's up to you to figure out *how* to reach them and get through to them. They might play on the team for different reasons, so it's up to you as the coach to figure out their *why* and make it worthwhile for them and their teammates."

My dad, the sage...

For the next two weeks, I watched each girl on the team. I could reach the competitive ones easily. I'd compete with them and make sure we did drills where they were engaged and challenged. I had a harder time with the quiet ones. I had to stay late with one girl after her ride didn't show up after we got back from an away game, and we had a heartbreaking chat that offered some insight into what was going on with her.

I learned she a foster kid who bounced around a bit and was having difficulty adjusting to life in school. My heart snapped in half when she looked at me and away and asked quietly, "does it get any better?"

I swallowed. "What? School? Life?"

"Both,"

"I, uh," I started but honestly had no idea what to say. "It does," I said even though I didn't know if it would. "You just need to find the right group of friends, and things will click for you. You can't go wrong with the nice kids. Just find a group of them and see what happens."

"People don't like me very much."

I sat there at a loss for words. My stomach clenched, and I desperately searched my brain, unsuccessfully, for something to say.

"I'm fine." She said after a minute. "Things are just hard right now."

I imagined that her "hard" was more complicated with her history and home life than most. And her "right now" was probably longer than most.

I looked over at her and bumped her shoulder with my own.

"I don't really know what to say. But if you ever want to talk or need help, just let me know. Just let me know." I repeated lamely.

God, please. Please don't ever let my future children feel this lost.

Actually...please just let me have future children, and I promise I'll love them through everything life throws at them. Just let me have them.

She smiled faintly at me and looked back towards the road. After ten minutes, we hit the ball back and forth. After another five minutes, she asked to borrow my phone to call her foster mom again. No answer. After another ten minutes of playing, her foster mom flew into the parking lot, tires squealing. She rolled down her window and bit out, "Sorry, she didn't tell me I needed to pick her up tonight."

"It's fine. We were just hanging out and hitting the ball around," I deflected. The girl looked up at me, gave a small smile, and loaded her stuff into the back of the van. She didn't look at me again as they drove away.

My heart broke for her.

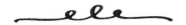

"What are your thoughts about being a foster parent?" I asked Josh over dinner that night.

"We can't take in your girl, Ash,"

"Not what I meant, dear," I grounded out.

He looked at me with a facial expression that screamed, 'you're not fooling me.'

"What I mean is, what if we can't have kids? We've been trying for over a year, and nothing's happened. If you're under thirty, you should get pregnant within the first year of unprotected sex. We've been doing that for about a year and a half now, and nothing! What if we can't have kids?"

"I'm sure there is nothing wrong with you." He assured me with blind faith. "Maybe we're just not timing everything right and missing the window."

"How can we be missing the window?" I exclaimed. "We're doing it all the freaking time! It's frankly exhausting."

And it had been. Peeing on the ovulation sticks wasn't accomplishing a whole bunch. Because my periods were so irregular, I was burning through many sticks every cycle while trying to pinpoint when I was ovulating. The trend the last few months had me seeing darker ovulation lines for a couple of days and then starting my period a couple of days later. But the line never got darker than (or even as dark as) the control line on the stick. I didn't know how to interpret that. Naturally, I used the internet to look up what that could mean because I was a researcher. But it wasn't helpful. Was I even ovulating? Was I ovulating for several days? Was the fact that I had my period a couple of days later causing me to shed any uterine lining that was supposed to be staying inside so a cute little embryo could snuggle up and make it home? That's why I wasn't getting pregnant. My mind was spinning.

I called the doctor's office when we hit the one year of trying to schedule an appointment, but the nurse didn't seem concerned. The earliest time they would give me to come in and see her was a couple of months out, hence why I was now starting to seriously stress that we were almost a year and a half into this TTC business, and I still hadn't seen a doctor yet. My first appointment was next week, and I was more than ready to get some answers. My mind was tormenting me with all the what-ifs.

What if something was wrong with me? What if something was wrong with Josh? What if we couldn't get pregnant? What if I got pregnant but had a miscarriage? What if I didn't get pregnant this month? Theoretically, I only had twelve chances per year to get pregnant. One ovulation per month, twelve months per year. Twelve. Yikes, that was a small window. What if one of us lost our jobs again? What if, what if, what if? My mind just wouldn't stop.

To make matters worse, it seemed like every one of my closest friends was getting pregnant just by drinking the town water. I had friends, cousins, and old classmates popping out babies like it was the forties, and their significant others had just returned from the war! I was happy for them... initially. And then it started to change. Their luck at getting pregnant started to wear on me. It started to make me overly conscious of the fact that they were getting pregnant, sometimes by accident, and I couldn't, no matter how often we tried. The happiness started to turn into bitterness and a little bit of anger. I stuffed it down inside; it wasn't their fault that I was struggling to get a BFP (big fat positive). Being unhappy at their baby news was foolish and immature of me. But I couldn't help those pangs from beating through me. I realized it was stupid. I recognized it was as foolish as being on a diet but being mad because someone else ate a cookie–it didn't affect me even a little bit, so I should feel nothing but joy for them.

But I wanted a cookie too...

"You have your appointment next week, and the doctor will let you know what's going on, so there's no use panicking or freaking out about this. We have loads of time. We're still young."

That was typical Josh. Don't worry, don't borrow tomorrow's problems today, don't research, and overwhelm yourself with all the possible scenarios of things that could be wrong... I probably should have tried adopting that mentality.

"I know, I know, I know. I just want to be prepared with questions. From everything I've read, I think I know the next steps and the expectations from those tests, so I feel well-prepared for everything the doctor says. But still. I just want answers. But! In the meantime, how do you feel about foster kids?" I jumped back to my original question.

"Obviously, I'd like to see if we could have our own biological kids. But I'm not opposed to foster kids. I don't really know much about it, though, to be honest."

"I've been doing some research -" I started.

"Naturally," he interrupted with a smile on his face as he forked in a glob of chicken parmigiana.

"I've been doing some research," I began again while staring him down. He smiled bigger. "The goal of the foster program is to return the kids to their parents. It's not to give them a safe, forever home. So that's a bit of a tricky part. I have to look into it some more, but it's an option if we can get placed with a kid who's up for adoption."

"What's wrong with adoption in general?"

"Oh my god, totally nothing. I just hadn't gotten there yet. I just dove into researching fostering first because of the girl on the team this year. Adoption research is next up on my list."

"Ahh, I see," he forked in another mouthful.

"So, how do you feel about it?"

"I told you, I don't really know much about it. So let's wait till next week to see what's going on before going there."

"Okay. So, how do you feel about adoption?" I pivoted.

"But you said you hadn't looked into that yet!"

"Well, I haven't. Perse. I know a little. I mean, my mom was adopted. And my aunt and uncles. And you have some aunts and uncles that were adopted. So obviously, it's crossed my mind."

Josh's family was mixed. His mom's parents had several of their own biological children and adopted several others. Josh never knew many of the details around the adoptions, though. Just two of his aunts were biological siblings that were adopted together.

My mom's parents had adopted all four of their children from different places. From what I understood, my grandfather had a medical condition that he didn't want to risk passing on to their children. Also, from what I gathered, they were all closed adoptions. My mom was around two years old when she was placed with my grandparents, but she had vague memories of her foster mom, that had her before that. My grandparents adopted my aunt from Columbia (the country), which I always thought was super cool. She was around seven-year-old and didn't speak a lick of English. She still has siblings in Colombia and kept in touch with them over the years. My mom always said that when her sister finally learned English, that my aunt told the best Colombian ghost stories.

I missed my grandma and wished she was still around, but she died a year before our wedding. I never wanted to talk to her more than when we had fertility issues or when I had adoption questions. I would have opened to her in a heartbeat. She would have completely understood the 'hole' inside me and the fear that I'd never have a child to love.

"Again, I'd like to see what the doctor has to say next week and then see what happens."

"Yeah, I see that. But what if- "

"Ash." Josh stopped me.

"What?" I whined.

"Just pump the brakes. We can talk about this all next week *after* your appointment, okay?"

I felt my face get hot and my heart race. Usually, I loved Josh's calm demeanor. It balanced out my high-strung personality. But right now, I *needed* him to talk through this with me. I was feeling lost, scared, and alone, and I wanted him to talk this out!

"But, Josh- "I started again.

"Nu-uh, nope. I'm not talking about this until after your appointment. I love you, and there's no one else I'd rather spend my life with, but I don't want to talk about this until we know for sure that something is wrong with one of us. Because I don't think that there is anything wrong, I think this topic is just acting as another way of stressing you out. I will not help you do that to yourself. There's no one else I'd rather give shit to," he smiled at me softly, "but I don't want to do it in a way that hurts you, and this conversation is just that."

I stared at him. I said nothing, though every cell of my body was itching to make me say something, to push the issue, to assuage my curiosity for answers. I fought it. He wasn't feeling the aching emptiness that being unable to have a kid was doing to me. He wanted kids, absolutely. But he didn't have that hole in him that was growing by the month. I didn't have any friends that were struggling with getting pregnant. I hadn't even told my friends that we were TTC. I was initially planning on it being a surprise announcement. I had Pinterest board after Pinterest board full of pregnancy announcement ideas. Now I had a Pinterest board (that was private) that had infertility memes on it and TTC advice. How much I had changed.

"Okay," I said after a minute.

"I love you." He added softly.

"I know. Love you too."

Seven

I PULLED THE DOOR open with a big exhale and entered the waiting room. I surreptitiously looked around while slowly approaching the windowed reception desk. The receptionist gave me the universal finger for 'wait a minute' as she finished her phone call. I hovered in front of her until she was ready to check me in, and then I found a seat in the corner. It was an early morning appointment, and the waiting room was empty. It didn't prevent me from feeling awkward. I opened my list of questions again and re-read them for the hundredth time. As I came across infertility stories and experiences on my various TTC apps, I made notes of symptoms, tests, and diagnoses. What if we can't have kids? What if something's wrong with me? Worry and fear became my constant companions.

On my sheet of paper, I had reminders to myself to make sure I asked about the likely suspects: am I ovulating, blood levels, polyps, was I on birth control for too long, etc. As the nurse opened the door in front of my seat, I shoved the wrinkled mess of a paper back into my purse and was escorted into the assessment room.

As she asked the standard questions and took my weight and height, I could feel my stress level rocketing. On the walls were pictures of pelvises, babies in utero, and happy moms and dads. There were pamphlets for smoking cessation, domestic abuse, diabetes, birth control methods, infertility, and more.

I pulled my eyes away quickly as the doctor knocked briskly on the door and entered the room.

"Hi Ashley, it's been a while." She started as she dragged the rolling stool over to the computer monitor. "So you're here today because you've been trying to get pregnant, but no luck yet?"

I nodded.

"Alright, let's see." She scrolled through some notes on the screen and then nodded to herself as her lips moved silently. "Okay, so tell me what's been going on."

"Well," I began. "I got off the pill a couple of years ago, and my husband and I have been having unprotected sex for the last year and a half but still no luck."

"Any notable family history for either of you? Any infertility,"

"Nope."

"Procedures, surgeries, or accidents that aren't in your file?"

"Nope."

"Are you a smoker?"

"Nope."

"How much do you drink?"

"I don't."

She glanced over from her computer screen when she checked the thing off and raised an eyebrow at me.

"I don't. I never really have. Growing up in a family of alcoholics stopped me from ever really getting into it." I shrugged.

"Drug use?"

"None," I affirmed again, sounding like a broken record. "I'm boring, I know."

"You call it boring; some others might call it healthy," she murmured while making a note on the computer.

"Have you been timing your cycles?"

"Yes, I have a couple of different app trackers, and I've been using the Ovulation Predictor test strips, but they give me weird results, so I don't know if it's operator error, a cheap brand, or what."

"What have you been seeing?"

I explained the results that I had been getting and how close I was getting the ovulation lines to the start of my next period. Over the last few months, the trend showed my darkened peak lines like four days or so before my period usually started, which was odd.

"Okay, so I want to run some different tests. First, I want to schedule a pelvic ultrasound and see what we're dealing with in there. I want to time that depending on where you are in your cycle so we can coordinate that when you check out. I also see a note in your file that your mom has Hashimoto's disease. A lot of time, thyroid problems can arise when you're older or become pregnant. So I also want to test your TSH levels to see where your thyroid is to ensure something hasn't developed since the last time we tested it. I want to run a couple of other blood tests as well. The other main one will be a test on your prolactin levels. High or low prolactin levels can affect ovulation, so let's see if that's off, and we'll go from there. Questions?"

Only about a million...

But I said, "No, that's mostly what I expected." I pulled out my crumbled sheet of paper and unfolded it. "We don't need to get an HSG or schedule an appointment for Josh's boys to be examined? Also, do you think there's an issue with my egg viability or reserve?" I picked my biggest questions that hadn't been addressed yet.

"Let's not schedule an HSG yet. Given your notes and you asking, I'm assuming you've read about it?" I nodded. "Then you know it's not a fun procedure, so if we can avoid it, let's do that. Also, I find it's a female issue more often than not, so let's get the simple tests for you out of the way first, then look at him."

"Oh," I repeated. I looked down at my list and looked up again. "So, my egg status?"

"I'm not worried about that at all. You're young, and you're healthy. I'd be surprised if there were an issue with your egg viability or the quantity, but if we strike out on the other tests, we can get you set up to get that looked at, but I don't think it will get that far."

I exhaled. "Okay then, I guess we'll start there."

"I know it seems overwhelming, but if we can find an issue with these test results, then we'll have saved you a lot in additional poking and prodding. Let's just go from here." She explained more about the next steps and what she'd be looking for, and I nodded along. I had expected this result. I knew I wasn't going to get answers today. And I guessed which tests would be ordered. But each day that went by felt like another missed opportunity.

"Remember to stop by the front desk to schedule a follow-up and to do your billing confirmations, and we'll give you a shout when you should come back for bloodwork."

I reviewed the visit and my next steps as I left the clinic. I certainly didn't think she would be able to produce an answer for me right then and there, but it was frustrating that they couldn't do the tests the same day. The rational part of me understood the reasons why. But the impatient person of me was screaming her frustration. I stopped my car at the crosswalk to let a pedestrian cross and realized I had never looked at my summary and bill from checkout. I gave the receptionist my "bill me" answer when she asked if I wanted to receive a bill or pay now, so I didn't know what it cost for today's visit. I grabbed the paper while I sat there and took a quick look. Thirty dollars. That's not too bad. I didn't know whether it would count as a specialist visit. I'd have to make a note when I got home to remember to pay that when it came in.

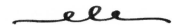

After scheduling my ultrasound and blood tests, I mentally prepared myself for getting poked with sharp, unpleasant needles. Something about needles going into veins sketched me out. So when the doctor called me back after my first round of blood tests and asked me to redo one particular blood test, I got squeamish but put my big kid shoes on and agreed I'd be in the next morning. The week had been busy but unfruitful. The ultrasound came back perfectly normal, with everything where it was supposed to be. Even my TSH levels for my thyroid were golden. However, my prolactin levels were elevated. She assured me that several things could have caused it. Sex, a too-tight bra, a cold, where I was in my cycle–all potential causes, so I shouldn't be alarmed. But I spent the rest of the night researching the causes and symptoms of elevated Prolactin levels, and to my mind, I found our infertility culprit! We finally found something to blame!

Fix my prolactin and say hello to baby!

So there I was. Six thirty in the morning and ready to be poked. Again. I had my pick of chairs in the empty waiting room and sat on the most comfortable-looking chair, though that wasn't saying much. The windowless room was bland; hospital white walls, thin brown-grey checkered carpet, and blue upholstered furniture. I tapped my foot to a fast rhythm while I waited for them to call my name. *What if we can't have kids? What if something more serious is wrong with me?* No. I told myself that this wasn't the case. My Prolactin levels were the reason for the wait, and everything would be cleared up soon.

I figured being the only person there would entitle me to a short wait time. But as ten minutes passed and no one called my name, I started to get antsy. Several other victims had checked in and left during my wait, and I was frustrated. I had to get to work. I didn't expect this to take forever, but now they were fifteen minutes late getting to me. I exhaled, not quietly, and looked at my phone again. After approximately twelve seconds (which, when you're impatient and nervous, feels like five minutes), I heard -

"Ashley! Hi! How are you?"

I put down my phone with a start and looked up. A family friend of my parents had lasered in on my location in the corner.

"Oh, hi." I lamely replied. In my defense, my mind doesn't work all that great before eight in the morning, and even then, it's by requirement, not because it wants to.

"How funny! I just saw your mom at the post office the other day!"

Ahh, the joys of small-town life.

"Small world," I said. Again, morning time was not my strong suit for making riveting conversation.

"How have you been? Your mom said you got a new job that's going well!"

"Yeah," I started. "My old firm's owner wanted to retire, and his son didn't want to take over. I ended up finding a new job that's closer to home, so that's been great. Plus, they let me coach field hockey, which has been super fun. Now, if I could just get Josh to have a job that wasn't almost an hour away, we'd be golden!" I smiled as I warmed up. Mornings may not be my strong suit, but who doesn't like to talk about themselves?

"What's new with you?"

"Same ol', same ol'." Betty smiled. "My daughter visited last weekend with the kids, so that was a blast. Her little guy is three, and the baby just turned a year. And," she lowered her voice conspiratorially, "she just told us she's pregnant again!" She mini-squealed.

Great. Someone else who's pregnant while I'm infertile-Myrtle over here.

"That's awesome! Congrats!" I felt my lips turn up. My voice gave the right pitch increase, but I realized I didn't feel it. Joy. I didn't feel happy for her. I should have. I should have felt happy for them. But all I felt was an overwhelming dread that that might never be me. Somewhere along the last year and a half, I lost my ability to be happy for others being pregnant. I wasn't even thirty, and here I was an infertile shrew? I chastised myself mentally and tried to build up some internal excitement.

"That's great." I semi-repeated, mostly to reaffirm it to myself. "Does she know what she's having?"

"She wants it to be a surprise again."

"I don't know how people can do that," I exclaimed. "I'd be desperate to get an idea so I could plan."

"When I had my kids, it was all the rage not to know and to let it be a surprise. I think that trend is coming back around. You'll see. You'll be the same way. You'll say that you want to know, and then you'll change your mind once you see those two pink lines!"

Her use of 'when' was maybe more of an 'if' at this point.

"Ashley?"

My head shot towards the door where a frustrated-looking phlebotomist was standing.

"Good seeing you. I'll see you later." I gave her a mini-wave as I stood up.

"Absolutely. And don't make your parents wait too long before having any grandchildren! Your mother mentioned she was sick of waiting!" She laughed out as a parting shot.

Gutted, my stomach turned, and I felt nauseous. I felt her words slice through me

A normally innocuous statement until you say it to someone staring down the infertility gun.

What if I can't have kids? What if I can't make Josh the incredible dad he was born to be? What if I never gave my parents grandkids? They 100% deserved to have grandbabies.

I smiled tightly and turned away. My heart raced and cracked a little more as her words settled in me. I followed the phlebotomist, rolled up my sleeve, confirmed my information, and re-lived her words repeatedly as the needle pierced my still-healing skin.

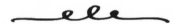

The clinic had called me the following day and scheduled an appointment for that afternoon, so for a third time that week; I made my way back into the hospital to talk with my doctor. The wait this time was nonexistent, and they brought me right back to see her.

"Okay, Ashley," she began. "Your bloodwork all came back relatively normal, as you know. Fortunately, you were at a point in your cycle that allowed us to draw blood immediately this week rather than making you wait a couple more weeks for a better-timed draw. However, as you also know, your prolactin level was high on that first test. I was hoping it was just a fluke thing, like I told you, but your level came back even higher on yesterday's test."

Naturally, I had researched this already on the off chance that this was my cause,' my reason, for not getting pregnant. I was on board with this being the culprit, hating my prolactin levels and cursing them till the day I died, but ultimately finding a medication that could fix them. Then have them fixed, get pregnant, and go back to our regularly scheduled programming of my planned-out life.

"Okay, so what next?" I jumped to the point.

She smiled somewhat grimly at me. "Well, we're closed most of next week because of Thanksgiving, but immediately after that, I'd like you to see our Endocrinologist. An elevated prolactin level can often show something going on with your hormones or glands. I talked with her this morning after I received your results, and she agreed to see you on the 29th. Do you have any free time that day?"

"Even if I don't have free time, I'll move some stuff around," I stated frankly but still politely.

"I figured as much. Here is some information from her office to look at in the meantime. I'm sure you'll use Dr. Google when you leave here but remember that this very well might not be something serious, so before you research something that freaks you out, try to keep an even head until you talk with Endocrinology."

Well, that sounded ominous.

As we said our goodbyes and she left the room, I looked back at the pamphlets lining the wall. My eyes fell on the 'Infertility' pamphlet that I had seen in what seemed like so many lifetimes ago.

And that's what this was, wasn't it?

Technically, I was infertile. Or maybe Josh was, but odds were more likely pointing at me.

The thought hit me like a ton of bricks.

I mean, I knew I was there because I couldn't get pregnant.

But seeing it defined by a small pamphlet in a doctor's office brought it home for me.

I was infertile.

***I** was infertile.*

Me, the girl next door. Voted smartest in the class superlatives. Runner-up for class clown. Perfect attendance, straight A's, never even received detention, Magna Cum Laude in college, and current CPA. Coach. Loving aunt, daughter, sister, wife. All boiled down. Infertile.

I might never be a mom.

I could get good grades. I could impress teachers, coworkers, or bosses. I could condition my body and mind, practice, and excel. I received offers to play field hockey and softball in college, damn it! I knew how to push my body and mind.

But I couldn't train for this. I couldn't make my body do this. No matter that I was hitting the gym daily. No matter that I was eating healthy. No work on my part could fix this. My own body couldn't get pregnant.

Over the years, I had heard various rants regarding fertility that my subconscious chose to haunt me with. Essentially, they all boiled down to several key themes. *Female bodies were made for this. Think of all the unplanned and unwanted pregnancies out there-it can't be that hard to get pregnant. Most of the people who can't get pregnant have treated their bodies so poorly that it's no wonder they can't have babies. If people can't afford the treatments, then they probably couldn't afford a child, anyway. Maybe infertility is God's way of saying 'it's not meant to be.*

Yup. Awful things to say.

Even so, those words lived rent-free in my mind. Rattling around, unwanted but ever-present. Casting doubt on my every decision and picking at every insecurity.

I thought I was made to be a mom. And my body was failing me. It couldn't do the *one thing* a female body was supposed to be able to do. What was the point of suffering through crappy periods every month if it didn't enable me to have a baby? People get pregnant by accident all the time! And I couldn't even get pregnant on purpose? What sick cosmic joke was this? Give a drug addict or an abuser an accidental pregnancy, but me? A healthy woman under thirty who didn't stay up past eleven if she could help it? Who had a stable job and a happy marriage?

Me?

I don't get a baby?!

My mind was reeling, and I felt like I was suffocating. As I stared at that pamphlet, I gulped in a breath, braced myself, and took a step towards it. I dragged it out of its plastic holder and stared without seeing the front page. I shoved it deep into my purse, turned around, and left the room—a heavy weight in my gut.

Eight

FOR THE NEXT WEEK and a half time seemed to crawl. I researched more (naturally) and found that elevated prolactin levels could indicate a prolactinoma—apparently a completely benign type of brain tumor. 'No big deal,' I read... yeah, right! A brain tumor is a brain tumor! My doctor's words of advice about not spiraling down a rabbit hole were ignored entirely in the face of possibly having a freaking brain tumor. I researched and read, found MRI pictures, and tried to self-interpret. Side note: I had literally no idea what I was looking at, but I still tried to decipher them. And above all else, during this time period, I drove my poor husband crazy. By the time my Endocrinologist appointment came, I had convinced myself I had a prolactinoma, and my husband was convinced that I was a nut job.

Sure enough, the doctor was quick and to the point at my appointment.

"You might have a prolactinoma. I'd like to get an MRI."

Boom. Done.

Not much of a bedside manner, but I appreciated the call to action to get this show on the road.

A rather expensive specialist visit just to be told that, but whatever, answers were answers. And we were on our way to getting them.

Even so, a wave of nausea rolled in and assaulted me. This was freaking terrifying. Every step. Every test. Every time they brought up something new, it scared me but also relieved a piece of me. I wanted an excuse so badly.

A reason. *Something, anything,* that could be assigned to our pregnancy delay and take the blame. Because then we'd have the problem identified, and we could set up a game plan of attack.

But... a brain tumor?

This was the first one that really, really scared me.

I left the hospital shaking, wanting to puke.

Even though I knew what they were going to say and suggest, it still hit different when coming out of the mouth of the doctor instead of Google. It made it more real.

It was the middle of the workday, but I still called my friend Megan just to freak out with someone. But when she didn't answer, panic hit. I had no one to talk to about this. I wanted to call my mom. I wanted my mom to tell me it would be all right.

My nose and throat burned with unshed tears, and my heart was racing with worry.

They said this type of tumor was benign...but what if mine wasn't?

What if something was seriously wrong with me, and we were coincidentally finding out because of the infertility testing?

I wanted my mom.

But I also didn't want to break the fertility issue news to her this way. That wouldn't be fair or kind. At this point, I wasn't expecting to be able to surprise her with a onesie that said 'world's best grandma' or a coffee mug with a cute saying on it as a way of announcing it. At this point, those dreams and plans had drifted through my fingers like water at the beach.

Even though I wanted to speak to my mom with a passion and fear that choked my breath and shook my entire body, I did the mature thing. I decided not to burden her with this. She had enough worries. She didn't need to add me and my infertility issues to the list.

The MRI was a little over a week later.

The small, but present, delay in scheduling had me gritting my teeth. Because once again, another delay was another missed month. Another negative test at home. But I pushed through my disappointment because this could be the answer that we had been waiting for. Finally, a light at the end of the tunnel!

My MRI was uneventful. I had to lie perfectly still for almost an hour while the machine whirred, clicked, and clacked above me. The technician played some soft country music hits into the booth, so that was a nice touch. But the entire time, I couldn't stop thinking that *this* was it. This was going to give us the answers that we needed.

Maybe.

Hopefully.

"We'll have the on-call doctor take a look sometime over the next few days and send your results." The technician said.

"Did you see anything that would be cause for concern? Should I have my husband near me when I take that call?" I tried to weasel a hint out of him.

"I can't make that call. I don't interpret the pictures. I just make sure they're clear for the doc. You'll have to wait for the call."

"But, like... was there anything super obvious there that I should be concerned about?" I pushed again.

He looked down his nose at me with a mini-scowl, and I took the hint—no answer from the tech. Stop fishing. Understood loud and clear.

After striking out with the technician, I compulsively checked the patient portal to see if someone had uploaded my results yet. Nothing was uploaded by the time I received a call back to the office a couple of days later, so I was more than ready to hear some answers.

And slightly worried. What if they didn't call with the news because it was really bad news? What if something was seriously wrong and they wanted to tell me in person?

I had convinced myself that I had a prolactinoma and that it was the cause of all my heartache, so I was relieved but nervous to finally head in for my appointment and get our next steps. Therefore, I was shaken when I came in for my second meeting with Endocrinology, and she said I didn't have one.

"What do you mean?" I repeated.

"You don't have a pituitary adenoma. Your scan was clear. You don't even have a little one. Though, I guess a super small one that we can't see could exist."

"But then, why do I have high prolactin levels?"

"It could be a couple of different things, but a prolactinoma isn't one of them. Because your levels are elevated, it might affect your conception goals. I want to get you started on a prescription called Bromocriptine. I only want you to take half a pill a day, but I think that will be enough to get your levels back in line with where they should be. In a little bit, I want you to get your blood retested to confirm, but for now, I'm going to hand you back to Dr. Bradlee, and she can take you from here."

As I stopped by the receptionist's desk to get my prescription called in, I wondered what could cause my high levels. I didn't get much further in my research than the possible brain tumor, as it seemed to be the most common reason. If this prescription fixed my levels and got me pregnant, then maybe the reason for the high levels was a moot point. Or 'moo point,' as Joey Tribbiani would say. As long as the prescription lowered my levels and let me get pregnant, I guess I didn't overly care.

As I called Josh and gave him an update, I drove by the pharmacy and picked up my new prescription. He was equally relieved that there was no tumor rattling around by my brain, but I could tell he was also getting frustrated.

"Could it be me?" He asked.

"I guess it could, but I figured that wasn't likely given how fertile your family is in general. Plus, Dr. Bradlee said nothing about testing you for anything. She seems to think it's me."

"Makes sense. It could be you if your hormone levels were off, but were they *that* off?"

"I don't know. I'm not a doctor," I bit back, letting my frustration leak a little.

"Well, maybe I'll schedule an appointment with my doc and see what he says. That way, we can stop wasting time and attack this from both ends."

"That's probably a good idea." I agreed. "Hold up. The hospital is calling back. I hope they didn't give me the wrong test results!"

Josh chuckled darkly, "that only happens in movies. See you after work. Love you, bye."

I switched over the line, "hello?"

"Hello, is Ashley there?"

"Yeah, that's me."

"Yes, this is the nurse from Dr. Bradlee's office. She just got a note from Endocrinology that you'll be moving back to her for your care, so she asked me to call you and to get a hysterosalpingogram, or an HSG, scheduled for you. Did Dr. Bradlee go over what that was?"

"Yeah, we had talked about it, and I had researched it a bit."

She explained anyway, "It's just an X-ray of your uterus and fallopian tubes to make sure that there aren't any blockages that might be blamed for your inability to get pregnant." I feel like she didn't listen to my response.

"I-"

She interrupted me.

"So, how does right before Christmas sound?" I heard people talking in the background and her murmur, "one moment, please."

"Yes, I'd like to get this done as soon as possible."

"Well, this test is cycle-specific, so we need to know the start date of your next cycle."

"Oh jeez, I've never been very predictable... when I checked it last night, my ovulation tracker app said I should be starting my period sometime around the sixteenth, but that could be off by seven days. I never really know."

"Let's go off with that, and if it changes, let us know. Also, how many days does your bleeding last?"

"That's also a tough question." I hedged. "Some cycles it lasts three days, other times it lasts seven."

"Well, this is certainly a challenging one. Let's make some assumptions and schedule you for ten on the twenty-second. And if your menstrual cycle is wonky this month, or you get pregnant, let us know." I wondered briefly about the chances of getting pregnant within the next couple of weeks. "You'll want to take some ibuprofen fifteen to thirty minutes before the procedure and bring a pad just in case you bleed or leak after. Also, let us know if there is any change to your insurance or billing in the meantime."

I quickly pulled my phone away from my ear and checked the calendar to ensure it would work. If not, I would make it work. "Yes, I can do the twenty-second at ten," I added it to my phone as a reminder.

"Great! We'll call the day before to remind you and to tell you where to go once you get into the clinic."

"Alrighty, "I agreed, "thanks!" I said chirpily, now grasping onto the new hope that maybe it's just a blocked fallopian tube. Yea, I thought to myself. A blocked fallopian tube seemed like a probable cause. It sounded like something that could be fixed easily enough. We could do this. This time, on this test, we'd have our answer.

I'm not infertile. I *can't* be.

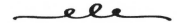

After the brain tumor debacle, a girl was only expected to take so much. I had so much turmoil built up inside me that I let our TTC cat out of the bag to someone other than my closest friends. So this brought my inner circle count up to four. I had my co-worker-turned-friend, Megan, as a confidant. My best friend from high school, Alaina. My softball friend, Lisa, and now a semi-friend, semi-acquaintance, Jamie.

A couple of days before my HSG, Josh and I were sitting at Mark and Lisa's house, watching Karli swing on the monkey bars. Our mutual friends, Jamie and Chris, were sitting with us. As the husbands went off to man the grill (because it required all three of them), Chris looked to Jamie, mouthed, "I want one," and left the porch. Jamie then turns to us and tells us how they're going to try for a baby sometime soon. She said that they were waiting for a little bit because Chris had just started his own company and Jamie was a teacher, so she wanted to time her maternity leave during the summer. As someone who had firsthand experience with trying to 'plan' when maternity leave would happen and how that backfired on us, I sprung to action to share my experience and recommendation on not to wait.

I broke down about how, initially, the plan was to have a baby anytime that *wasn't* tax season, so I wouldn't have to miss the main part of my year. But then, after a year of trying, you wonder if the timing is so important - maybe it's more important to just be able to get pregnant. I had a mini rant about how it's ridiculous that you must wait for the one-year mark to pass before getting help if you're under thirty. I told her about all our struggles, the tests, and the waiting game. *Everything*. By the time I was done, Lisa and Jamie were staring at me wide-eyed and completely thrown by the intensity of my reaction and experiences. And as I was wrapping up my diatribe, I realized what I was doing: offering unsolicited advice on someone else's conception plans; I was being a total hypocrite! I apologized for coming off so strong and sounding so 'preachy.' But she assured me it was good to talk about this with someone because she would have hated to have tried for two years, to no avail, and then have to wait another two years for answers. Now she knew to be proactive.

After we left for the day, I realized that I had shared details I hadn't shared with anyone else. And it was a bit therapeutic to get that off my chest. I also felt like I could impart some, shall we say, *wisdom* to someone who was always fed the same line I was. That cautionary line being: 'always use protection or you'll get pregnant.' For the first time, I wondered if I was doing a disservice to others by not discussing this more. Maybe others are just like me, struggling, and perhaps if we all talked about this more, then they wouldn't feel so alone. Why was talking about infertility so taboo?

Was it because of the insensitive comments that people everywhere make without even realizing it? Was it fear of judgment? A judgment about something we had no control over. Fear of pity? I didn't know, but it was time for some soul-searching.

I also wondered if I had scared her half to death and if I maybe should have been more positive.

Nine

As I walked into the radiology department, I cursed myself for researching HSGs so thoroughly. Yesterday when the nurse called me, she gave me the same description and outlined the same expectations that the nurse had a couple of weeks ago: expect mild discomfort, take ibuprofen or acetaminophen, and bring a pad. She tacked on that I might want someone to drive me just in case I was shaky after the procedure, but that seemed overdramatic. Plus, we were still keeping the whole infertility testing under wraps, so it's not like I could ask my mom to just drive me to and from the hospital for a 'procedure' and not talk to her about it.

Honestly, not talking to her about any of it was killing me.

When they told me I might have a brain tumor, it shook me. During this whole process, I felt very alone. Adrift. My well-thought-out plans for a cute pregnancy announcement dried up and shriveled into dust. The comments about 'you've waited long enough,' 'there's never a right time,' 'there will always be debt,' etc., were wearing on me. And I didn't want to come out and say we were unsuccessfully trying because then it just brought up more questions. And I had enough questions of my own! I didn't need someone asking me why we couldn't get pregnant. Or if we tried this position. Or if we were doing our timing right. Or if I was using ovulation predictor kits. How long we had been trying and how it would happen once I stopped trying and stressing about it. Or how his/her cousin's best friend has a sister who had a neighbor who got pregnant with twins after... Or enjoy your sleep while you can!

Or someone foolish saying, "well, trying is the fun part!"

Because no...

No, it fucking wasn't.

There was no fun part anymore.

Timing sex with ovulation days was exhausting. There was a ton of pressure. It was straining our relationship. Not in a 'this is going to break us up' sort of way. Just in an 'I literally can't get in the mood' sort of way. I stopped telling Josh when I was possibly ovulating because it seemed to stress him out. However, he could always tell after the fact, given that I would lie on my back with my feet up in the air over my head, trying to help those little buggers the best I could—no gravity barrier when they were trying to make their way to my wonderful little egg. We tried Pre-Seed for a while as a lubricant that was supposed to act as a superhighway for the sperm to travel on. Obviously, no luck with that. But we tried.

Karli's mom, Lisa, told me about how her sister tried for years to get pregnant but then had to rely on IVF. And that was ten years ago. It shocked me into remembering once again that one in every seven couples experiences infertility and that you never really know who has experienced it because no one talks about it. She promised me that her sister would be more than happy to talk to me about it, but I assured her I wasn't at that point yet. I wasn't ready to talk to someone I didn't know about all this. And especially about IVF. I wasn't so sure it would get to that point for us.

But then again, that conversation was several months, blood draws, ultrasounds, and MRIs ago.

Now was a different story.

Maybe I should circle back with her... The possibility was frightening. I was ashamed, to say the least. Looking back at it all now, I wish I had been more vocal and shared with my family sooner. Or maybe looked for an in-person infertility support group. It would have helped to hear my pain through someone else's voice.

I found a great community online on different fertility forums that I used to solicit support and ask questions. And those people became 'my tribe' (I don't mean that in a cultural appropriation way). I was on those apps daily, checking in on my 'friend's' results and the latest procedures. Just like they were doing with me. But there was still something to be said for not having my mom, dad, or brother in the loop and not being able to call on them for emotional support.

As an X-ray tech escorted me from the waiting room, I mentally prepped myself. Everything I had read online had said that this procedure had the potential to become quite... Unpleasant. I changed into my johnny, hoping that the Advil I had taken earlier was enough to make this not so bad. Probably a fool's hope, but a hope.

I hopped up on the table and sat gingerly. The crinkly paper scratched my legs, and the overhead light was almost blinding. The technician came over with a clipboard, asked me some standard questions, and handed the clipboard to me to sign.

"Is there a chance you could be pregnant?"

I inwardly grimaced. "Not likely," I assured her.

"Okay," she turned and headed back to the station that held the computer. Meanwhile, the radiologist came in and came straight to me.

"Ashley, I'm so sorry. I saw the name but didn't realize it was you. The married last name threw me. Do you want me to get someone else? I don't want you to be uncomfortable."

Small town life strikes again.

As luck would have it, apparently, Dr. Nicholson was the radiologist working today. She was very close to my best friend's family. But I didn't think for a minute that she'd go and talk about doing an HSG on me with anyone. So her concerns were thoughtful but unnecessary. Plus, there was no way I was going to ask for another doctor now-especially if I meant I had to delay this test.

"Nope, no problem! I'm totally fine with you!"! I assured her absently, hoping my vagina didn't look weird compared to other people: a weird thought to have, but whatever.

"Are you sure? I don't mind getting another doctor."

"Totally, absolutely fine!" I promised.

"If at any point you feel differently, let me know." She waited for my nod and then went on to quickly overview what she was going to be doing: having me lay back, prying me open with the ducky lips, using a balloon to inflate my cervix, sticking a power washer with fluid up into my uterus, and then setting that puppy on high (my unflattering summary). Meanwhile, the x-ray machine would take images. The hope would be that a blocked tube would appear in the pictures, and we could go from there. However, there was a chance that pushing fluid into my uterus and through the tubes would inadvertently cause any blockage to break. So it might not show that there was a blockage because the process of this test might clear it during the actual procedure.

"So, let's get started!" She smiled at me reassuringly, "and again, this can sometimes be... Uncomfortable. So, if you need me to stop at any point, just let me know."

I nodded, gingerly put my feet in the stirrups, preserving my modesty until the last possible second, and laid back on the cold table.

Actually, the entire room was a little chilly.

Dr. Nicholson redirected the light down to my coochie and asked me to slide my butt closer to her so it was along the edge of the table. I arched and inched close to her, feeling a little mortified that she now just had a full face of my vagina, but trying to mentally remind myself that she's a doctor and to ignore the awkwardness.

As Josh always says to me: it's only awkward if you let it be awkward.

I don't always agree with that. But it served my purpose here, so I was willing to go with it for peace of mind.

"Okay, so I'll be inserting the speculum now."

She gently inserted it, and I grimaced slightly as she gently cranked it wide.

"You okay?"

"Yup," I took a deep breath.

"Try to relax and loosen your muscles."

I nodded—every fiber of my being focused on the cold metal inside me, stretching me uncomfortably.

"Okay, now I'm going to insert the balloon to open your cervix,"

Oh my God!

"Ow," slipped out.

"I know, I know. I'm having trouble inserting it. Just hang in there. Let me know if it gets to be too much."

I started deep breathing.

"Try to relax. You're doing great." A small pause. "Okay, I'm in. I will be opening your cervix so the catheter can come through. You might feel some cramping now."

Holy crap!

Ouch.

"Oh my God," I gasped out.

"You're doing great," she said placatingly. She definitely did this a time or two in the past. She knew exactly what I was going through. There was a gentle calm in her voice.

The whole cervix being opened piece was tricking my body into thinking it was in labor. My uterus started contracting and cramping in response. It wasn't pleasant.

"Okay, here comes the dye. Almost done."

"Oh my God. Oh my God. Oh my God."

My back arched off the table of its own accord. My feet dug into the now-warm stirrups. Tears started pooling out from my clenched eyelids and down my cheeks. All my attention was on the pain. They said it could be uncomfortable. They didn't say it would hurt like this

Dr. Nicholson looked up at me in concern. "Do you want me to stop?"

"No, just... Just finish it." I half cried half grunted out.

"Almost done," she murmured distractedly. "All set!"

As she pulled the catheter out, deflated the balloon, and removed the instruments from me, I couldn't stop shaking. My legs felt weak, and I had fingernail prints edged into my palm from squeezing my hands so hard. My uterus was still cramping in reaction to the violation that had just occurred, and I wanted to crawl up into a ball and wallow.

A tissue appeared in front of me.

Dr. Nicholson patted my back and had a second tissue ready for me after I soaked the first one.

I took a calming breath and braced myself. "So what's the verdict? Am I blocked?"

"No, honey. Everything looked perfect. Your uterus looked normal, and the tubes were clear. Of course, there's a chance we dislodged something when pushing the dye through. But I don't think that's the case."

I sat there... *Stunned,* staring at the rolling computer cart next to me.

Another strikeout.

Another dead end.

"Here, let me help you down."

Help me down? Heck. I wasn't even close to being done with processing. Numbly and shakily, I took her hand and stepped down. I immediately felt wet seep out of me.

"Did you remember to bring a pad, or do you need me to get one for you?"

"I have one," I murmured distractedly.

"Okay, I'll leave you to get changed. I'll get everything over to Dr. Bradlee today so she can call you on the next steps." She smiled softly at me and exited quickly. She said her goodbyes and post-procedure warnings and took her leave.

I stood there for a minute, staring blankly at the room in silence.

Pure silence echoed in my head.

I felt it would be much easier to stomach this inability to conceive if we had something to blame. A culprit. A reason. All this unknown was killing me. I just wanted to have a reason why we couldn't get pregnant. Because if you know 'why,' then you either have something you can work towards fixing, or you have something that can't be fixed and you can move on. This in-limbo state was torture.

The room swam before me. I blinked hard and cleared my throat.

What if we could never have kids?

I tried to rally. To remove myself from the downward spiral, I could feel hovering over me.

Okay, what was the next step?

Oh jeez. I had no idea. I never even thought I would get this far without answers. I was healthy! Why couldn't I get pregnant?

What could be next?

How much more of this could I take?

Ten

I RECEIVED A CALL that afternoon from Dr. Bradlee recapping the HSG findings and asking me to come in for progesterone bloodwork in the first week of January. She said that the test would help her determine if I ovulated. She also had me schedule an appointment with the administrator after she got off the call.

"Okay, so bloodwork on the third, and you'll see Dr. Bradlee on the 18th at one forty." she summarized. "No changes to your insurance or address?"

"Nope, all the same." I felt like I was always confirming this question.

"We'll bill you after everything has gone through insurance, per usual."

"Sounds good," I muttered into the phone as I checked emails on my work computer.

"Great, we'll see you then!" Then she hung up.

The next few days flew by as Josh, and I prepared ourselves for all the Christmas festivities.

By the time we got to my parent's house on Christmas evening for dinner and presents, I was emotionally and physically spent.

I usually loved Christmas time.

I adored family gatherings. I loved presents (both giving and receiving, though mostly receiving), the food, and the excitement.

But last Christmas, as Josh and I were opening presents, we looked up at each other and said, "this could be our last Christmas with just the two of us!" In naïve excitement.

Now that this second Christmas was here, we shared the same thought again this morning, but we also wondered if maybe it wouldn't be. If maybe we would have many more Christmases with just the two of us...

We were eating Christmas dinner in the dining room when a Sarah McLachlan-like commercial came on the tv in the other room. I had just spooned a heaping pile of mashed potatoes into my mouth when a voiceover could be heard from the other room.

"For just five cents a day, you can sponsor a child, like Josiah or Emily. For just five cents a day, you could save and change a life..."

This seemed innocuous enough.

Until my dad said, "Hey Mary, do you think they'd let us adopt a grandchild from them since Ashley and Josh refuse to give us one?"

Umm, what?

No.

No, he did not.

He did not just say that.

I couldn't believe it.

All the emotions that had built up in me over the last year and a half swallowed me. I slammed my spoon onto the table next to my plate. And I erupted.

"We're fucking trying, okay! We're trying! It's not working! This past month, I've been put through the wringer on all sorts of tests, including dealing with possibly having a freaking brain tumor!" I ended in a near-shriek. "I don't! But for a while, they thought I had one." I felt the tears burning, and my vision got wavy. I inhaled and kept going, much more calmly, "it's not working. Nothing is working. We. Are. Trying. But nothing is working, and nothing is going according to plan. And no one knows why!"

Their faces were aghast as they looked at me. Josh looked like he had just seen a car accident in real-time. My brother looked like he might laugh, and my mom was not far behind him. Only my dad looked like he believed me.

I was heavily breathing while staring them down when Josh reached over and started rubbing my back.

"Wait," my mom said after a beat, looking at both of us more critically. "Are you being serious?"

They all continued to look at me, and in order to not erupt into waterworks, I kept my lips pressed tight. I looked down at my plate and tried to stuff the emotions away.

"Josh?" my mom called.

"Yeah, no. That's all true. We've been trying. It hasn't... been good."

"Oh, my God." My mom breathed. She didn't look like she was laughing anymore. "Oh, my god."

Josh soldiered on, "well, on that cheerful note..." he speared a piece of turkey with his fork and took a bite. He used his other hand to pat the back of my neck gently and gave it a firm squeeze. When I looked at him, he mouthed, "easy; I love you."

I looked back at my family and took in their reactions. My brother looked shell-shocked, his eyes still bouncing back and forth from Josh to me. My mom looked appalled and completely devastated. And my dad looked... broken.

"Sorry Ash," he whispered.

"I know. It's fine." Now that I had a minute to calm down, I was embarrassed I had lost it like that. "I know. I'm sorry. It just kind of built up." It wasn't their fault. They had no idea. And I went back and forth on telling them. But whenever I tried, it felt awkward, so I always deflected.

"How," my mom coughed uncomfortably. "How long have you been trying?"

"A year and a half," I replied while pushing sweet potatoes around my plate.

"Oh my god. Ash." My mom looked wrecked.

"You don't have a brain tumor?" My dad homed in on that tidbit of information.

"No, the MRI cleared me."

"Jesus." My brother swore, still looking aghast.

"Yeah," I sighed.

A little while later, as we were cleaning up, my mom cornered me and asked for more details.

Do they know why? How come you didn't tell me? What's next? When's your next appointment?

Then she surprised me with, "I wish you had told me. If I had known, I would never have allowed them to do the hysterectomy this summer. I would have carried a baby for you if it came down to that, honey. I offered it to my best friend years ago after your brother was born. I would have absolutely done the same for you."

"Mom, you're fifty. It wouldn't exactly be safe. Plus, you were having a ton of issues. You needed that surgery. It's not like it was elective."

"I could have just had them take out the ovaries and tubes. I could have asked them to leave my uterus if I had known, Ash!"

"I wouldn't ask that of you, Mom."

"You wouldn't have had to. I would have volunteered in a heartbeat. Same with if you needed an egg. Whatever you had needed, I would have given it to you."

And she would have.

I had the best mom.

"I know, Mom. I'm hoping we can figure something out before we get that desperate." Though honestly, I thought we wouldn't. I had been doing more research on fostering and adopting. One of my co-workers at work was just approved to be an emergency foster parent, so we were chatting about it the other day. I felt guilty for viewing foster parenting as my backup plan, though like a Band-Aid rather than stitches. Regardless, it wasn't the time to make that decision now. I was just keeping my options open and my finger on the pulse.

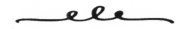

January rolled in, and it was nothing short of overwhelming. In a cruel twist of fate, I had not one but two baby showers to attend. One baby shower was for my sister-in-law and the other one for my best friend. My sister-in-law's shower was uneventful but depressing. Having each family member ask me when it was 'my turn' to have babies was difficult, to say the least.

Trust me, Auntie, I want it to be my turn too!

Instead, I repeated our catchphrase, "we're just trying to pay off some debt first," and smiled beatifically as if they didn't gut my heart out every time they asked or brought up the topic.

My best friend Alaina's shower was more of the same. Except there was a little bitterness to it on my end. It was painful because we had started softly trying around her wedding date, and here she was, celebrating a pregnancy that I had been trying to achieve for almost two years. I hated myself for feeling that way. But I couldn't shake it. Plus, dealing with the prying questions about when it was my turn was torturous. But as luck would also have it, I was sitting at a table next to Dr. Nicholson's, and if she overheard that question, she would lean over and interrupt.

Bless her heart.

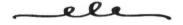

My husband had called his PCP right after Christmas and scheduled a generic physical to see if his doc had anything to add to our list of suspects. Fortunately, his doctor's office was able to fit him in quickly for the first week of the new year.

When he called to tell me what happened during his appointment, I almost drove off the road from laughing so hard.

"He asked me if I was ejaculating inside your vagina!" Josh roared with laughter.

"Say what now?" I needed more details because I was confused.

"I had my normal check-up. Weight, height, turn your head, and cough. Yada yada. And I told him we were trying for a baby, and you were being put through the wringer on all sorts of tests. So I asked if maybe my boys could be the reason, and we chatted a bit, and then he left the room. I'm just sitting there on the bed, contemplating taking a nap because, as you know, I can sleep anywhere, and he pops his head back in and clarifies to me, 'you're ejaculating *into* her vagina, correct?'! No joke!"

"Oh my god." I laugh. "You should have said 'no'! You should have said that you read that your chances of conception were higher if I swallowed it or something equally ridiculous!"

"What, like, I've been drawing ancient Mayan symbols of fertility on your lower back with my sperm?" He kept laughing.

"Exactly!" My eyes were watering.

"Well, I didn't think that fast. He caught me off guard. I just nodded and said 'yup,' and he shut the door again.

"Next time." I fake-comforted him with a smile

"Yeah," he agreed softly. "So anyway, he put in an order to the lab at the clinic to do a semen analysis done just to see if there were any red flags on my end. I'll head over there tomorrow and do the deed. He mentioned that sperm are sensitive to extreme temperatures, so I'll keep those little buggers insulated the best I can."

"I don't get the joke."

"What joke?"

"About temperature and keeping them insulated? You're saying you're going to wear two boxer briefs or something?"

"No, no, no. Sorry, I skipped a step. No, there's no room at the clinic to drop off my sample there. I basically have to go to the lab, get a cup, go home, do the deed into the cup, and then bring it back to them."

"Oh. Wouldn't it just be easier to use a room there?"

"I don't make the rules, dear." Josh chuckled.

"Yeah yeah, I know. It's just foolish to not have a private room for that kind of stuff."

"There must not be a need for it. Plus, I'm more than happy doing my part in the comfort of our own home. Just need to make sure that the ride back doesn't result in a car accident or some other delay that could damage the specimen."

I purred at him. "My, my, Doctor. You sound so knowledgeable." I smiled at my windshield as I spoke to him via car Bluetooth.

"You know it, baby." He purred back. "I'll see you tonight and give you a thorough physical. Doctor's orders."

I started laughing. "Okay, okay. I'll see you tonight. Love you."

"Love you too," he chuckled.

"Bye."

I hung up and thought to myself, 'there's no one else I'd rather be infertile with.'

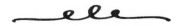

"Oh my god. Ash. Oh. My God."

It was the next day, and Josh had gone into the clinic that morning, and then it was radio silence while he did what he needed to do.

I made sure not to text him so as not to disturb the mood or any... culminations... that may or may not be occurring. So I let him reach out to me when he was done, which brought us to now.

"Oh no. What happened?" I braced myself for whatever ridiculousness was about to transpire.

"I just saw your dad."

"Okay?"

"Twice,"

"Okay?"

"I saw your dad twice," he repeated.

I waited.

"At the hospital. No. *Leaving* the hospital, actually. With my hand clutching a brown paper baggy like it had three kilos of coke and $50,000 inside." He let that sit.

"Is that a lot of coke?"

"Is that a lot of money?" He responded

"Okay, so he saw you with a paper bag that had your empty cup in it?"

"Yes!"

"Okay," I dragged out, not sure where these uncharacteristic dramatics were coming from.

"He obviously didn't see the cup, but he did eyeball the bag and then asked me if it was my lunch." He paused dramatically. "He knew it wasn't my lunch, Ash!"

I started laughing outright.

"Obviously, he was a little curious about what I was doing there. But after clumsily avoiding any prying questions, I got out of dodge and headed home. Then, once I finished my dirty work, I headed back to the hospital with the container secured between my bare stomach and the seat belt. I'm just trying to keep those guys, or girls, as warm as possible." He was really picking up speed now. I smiled as he got more into his story. My husband was adorable. "I swear to God it was about two degrees today."

"It was chilly," I murmured sympathetically.

"Chilly?" He exclaimed. "It was like the tundra out there. I know we're no Minnesota, but not a day you want to be walking around with a cup full of sperm. And!" He got worked up again. "All I could think was, 'I hope I don't get pulled over with a cup full of sperm in my shirt!"

Spittle flew from my mouth as he caught me off guard on that one. I had to wipe a tear from my eye, and then I worked on the spit that had landed on my computer screen.

"So then, who do I run into on my way back into the building to drop off my sperm sample? My father-in-law! Again! We crossed paths outside this time, and the whole time we were talking, all I was thinking about was the rapidly cooling sperm in my pocket. Now I would prefer not to see anyone I know when walking around with a container full of sperm, but I really don't want to see your dad. Nothing against your dad. But I'm doing you regularly so we can make a baby, and now he knows it, and I'm just walking around with a cup of jizz. So I don't want him asking questions about why I'm back at the hospital. Though I'm sure, he could take a guess."

"Oh, I'm sure he's got an inkling. But he wouldn't pry and ask questions. Now, if you ran into my mom... that's another story."

"What a day." Josh exhaled in my ear.

"That part is over now. One thing off your checklist. You can take a breather, dear." I tried for a calming tone because he seemed like he needed it.

"I mean, really. Your tests are awful, and mine is that I need to orgasm. I definitely got the easier tests. I'm not going to complain." There. That sounded more like my unflappable husband.

"That is totally funny you saw him twice, though. He went to visit my grandpa today. It must have just been super coincidental timing that he was arriving and then leaving when you were coming and going."

"Coincidental? More like a cosmic joke." He scoffed.

"Did they say when you'd get your results?"

"Nope, just more waiting."

"Bummer."

"Yeah," he agreed.

We both paused.

I broke it. "So what porn did you watch when you were doing it in the cup?"

"Got to go now, bye!"

Click and then silence.

I laughed, put my phone down, and got back to work.

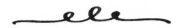

Ash," Josh moaned out.

"Yes, dear?" I chuckled in reply.

I was sitting at work, chipping away at another early tax return, and was eager to hear about Josh's latest drama. Now that Josh was involved in the infertility diagnosis process, it gave me a sense of freedom and levity in the situation that I didn't have before. It was a nice mental shift for me.

"Two things." He started. "One: when I was twelve, I broke my arm being stupid on the basketball court."

I waited. Josh was building up to another storytime.

"And when I broke my arm, my parents decided not to take me to our normal hospital forty-five minutes away, but the one closest to the school. Which is obviously *our* current hospital."

"Hmm," I murmured distractedly.

"But that was the only time I've ever gone to that hospital. In my life. Until I had to do the semen analysis yesterday."

"Josh, I'm working on a kind of tricky return right now. Can we talk about this later?" I tried to be supportive, but it was my first year on this client (technically all the clients, given that it was my first tax season there), so I wanted to give it my full attention.

"Wait a sec. I'm getting there. So anyway, I confirmed all my updated information with the lab yesterday, but apparently, none of it stuck. So they called today to discuss my semen analysis results."

Now he had my full attention. "And?" I asked with excitement.

"And..." he dragged out. "They didn't call *me*! They called the number they had on file from when I was twelve. Aka, my parents' house phone!"

"Are you kidding me?" I didn't know whether I should be horrified, worried, or find it funny. A part of me was nervous that his family now knew, and it wasn't us that told them. A part of me found the situation hilarious. This whole thing is like a comedy of errors.

"Yeah, so I get a call from my parents telling me they just got a call from the lab and that my results are in and would like to discuss them with me. They asked me what tests I had done and if something was wrong. I really didn't want to get into this with them, so I dodged and got off the call as soon as I could. But really! What are the chances?"

"Dear lord. This is a mini train wreck. If it wouldn't open such a can of worms, I say we should just come out to people. But I really don't feel like I can answer their questions without having a mental breakdown." I have been walking a tightrope of emotions lately. Very trigger happy.

"Understandable. I don't want to field questions either."

I sat back in my chair and looked out the window. My office was on the second floor, next to a beautiful pond. It was stunning to look at during the fall, but in the summer, it just made me jealous to see people outside enjoying the sun. In the winter, when it was covered by snow, it just served the purpose of making me squint whenever I looked outside.

"The good news, but also terrible news, is that I got my semen analysis results."

"Oh! Right!" I sat forward eagerly. "Tell me, tell me!"

"So, the results were not good, which is good. Because now we have the smoking gun! It turns out that the problem has been me. When I called the lab back, they said that a good value to have in a normal sperm analysis is anywhere from 40 to 100 million. I had less than 500,000. So, I'm totally shooting blanks!"

"That's awesome." I paused. "Well, not really... but you know what I mean!" The quest for The Reason was over!

"Naturally, they want me to come back and retest just to make sure, but I guess I need to wait a few days between samples, or the numbers get skewed. I should be able to get them a second sample sometime in the next two weeks, and we'll have another data point to add to our file!" That's my engineer–talking data points and evidence. God, I love him.

"Okay, that sounds promising, I think. But I do have a side question. Do they think that something is wrong with you? Like, are you okay? Does having that low of a count show that something serious might be wrong with you?"

"I'm not sure. I didn't ask. I didn't even think to ask that." He trailed off. Now, no doubt wondering if a low count indicated something to be concerned about.

"Okay, so you need to go back in a few days?"

"Yeah, but I think we finally have the start of our answers, dear!"

"Sounds like it," I agreed.

"I wish I had been tested earlier. It would have saved you from going through some crappy tests and would have gotten the ball rolling a little sooner."

"Water under the bridge. Now we know. That's all that matters. We certainly had no reasons to suspect you were possibly the driving force, so 20/20 hindsight and all that."

"Still," Josh said.

"Still," I agreed softly.

We said our goodbyes, and I got back to work. I had a return to finish.

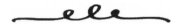

Even though the last month had been very busy, I still dreaded the wait until my follow-up with Dr. Bradlee. My research could only take me so far. I didn't know what our next steps would be—discovering that Josh's sperm count was low opened a new can of worms for us. However, this particular 'can' wasn't discussed all that much on the TTC apps and forums. High prolactin levels, ovarian cysts, thyroid issues, structural issues, Endometriosis, Polycystic Ovary Syndrome (PCOS), autoimmune disorders, and more—are all discussed on the apps. It made sense as most of the people on the apps were women. Of course, there were posts on male infertility, but it didn't seem to be a focus point, so I couldn't collect a lot of information from there. Josh just told me to wait to hear what the doctor had to say and then rolled his eyes at me. However, when his second test was only slightly better than his first (1.4 million), I wanted to educate myself the best I could so I could have a more meaningful discussion with the doctor when that time came.

I parked my car, grabbed my purse, and wound my way through the parking lot. Lost in my thoughts on how this appointment would go, I coasted through registration and up to the waiting room for Medical Team A. I checked my phone and saw a couple of 'good luck' texts from my inner circle of four. It still wasn't easy to talk about the conception woes that we were going through, but it was nice to have someone to whom I could vent. Jamie and Chris had taken the plunge and started trying as well. I guess my situation freaked her out a little. But she was still optimistic, and it had only been a month or so of trying. But my story freaked her enough that she was researching every possible thing that could go wrong so she'd be prepared. She also said she'd be demanding a visit with her OBGYN at six months rather than waiting until she hit a year. Since she is under thirty, I wasn't sure how that would work insurance-wise, but she was determined, and nothing I could say would change her mind. Another significant find since Christmas: my mom was an obsessive researcher. I decided that I received that trait from her. She dove into the reproductive waters like she was a Coast Guard Veteran. Her tablet received more use this last month than it had since she bought it years ago. It was to where she was getting conception ads from all the cookies she had gained during her searches.

It was nice to talk to her about my mental struggles and the depression fog I was battling. It seemed like it got a little harder each day, but I kept putting up the good fight.

I shot off some quick texts to my mom and friends, put my phone away, and glanced around the waiting room.

There were a couple of elderly patients and then a couple of patients between forty and sixty. I was by far the youngest person here. I felt that a lot hinged on this appointment, which increased my stress. I was projecting a calm demeanor, but under the surface, I was mentally all over the place.

They called me back and brought me to the room. I tried to brace myself mentally. I didn't think we would have good news today, so I wanted to be prepared.

I tapped my foot nervously as the nurse took my vitals and as the wait dragged on, I picked at my cuticles. A knock on the door caught my attention.

"Hi, Ashley. How are you?"

I hated that question.

"I'm fine. Getting worried that this will never happen to us. But fine."

"I understand. I'm sure all the waiting was wearing you down a bit. Especially after waiting for so long to be able to make an appointment."

Lady, you have no idea.

"Well, I'm sorry to say I don't have any good news for you." There it was. "Your bloodwork was unremarkable. The ultrasound was clear. Your uterus looked great. And your ovaries were an appropriate size. There was no free fluid. Your HSG was clear as well. Dr. Nicholson saw no blockages. The fluid could pass through without a problem, and there didn't appear to be any unusual topography that could influence a fertilized egg from taking root. Endocrinology found no evidence of a prolactinoma, so that was good news as well. Because even though they are always benign, it's never fun to think of having a tumor messing with your hormones. And, your bloodwork from earlier this month showed you did indeed ovulate, so we know that's occurring."

"Okay," I semi-asked, semi-confirmed while trying to get her to get to the crux of the matter.

"The lab downstairs copied us on his semen analysis results, both sets, and even though his numbers improved slightly on the second sample, it really looks to be a case of male factor infertility. I know we had touched on that possibility a few months ago, but it's usually only a third of the cases that we see, so we always like to rule out the female side first."

I darkly thought that maybe they should start with the men instead because even if it's not all that common, it seemed a hell of a lot less unpleasant. Plus, a lot cheaper. One semen analysis for us? $75. One MRI? Much more than that.

"So, I think we've done all we can with the resources available to us here at our hospital."

I blinked.

If you're amenable, I will get a referral to Dr. McBride over in Vermont. She's a board-certified OBGYN, but she also specializes in reproductive endocrinology. We refer many patients to her when they've spent all our resources here. She's an excellent doctor. I think you'll like her a lot. She is very compassionate, and she'll have a lot more specialized knowledge on what your next steps should be, especially with your husband's results being so out of normal range. You might need to do an Intrauterine Insemination or an IUI with his low numbers. But maybe something is blocking his duct-work, so to speak, that could be fixed, and then an IUI wouldn't be necessary."

"So," I dragged out. "Going forward, I'll no longer be seeing you, but I'll be seeing her? For everything?"

She seemed apologetic but nodded and affirmed, "that's correct."

"So, I will no longer be coming to this hospital. At all. Except to see my PCP when I need my inhaler refilled or for random strep throat tests? And now, anything conception related, I'll be seeing someone who is an hour away... in Vermont?" I wanted to confirm again because I wasn't super in love with this concept. Obviously, Operation Pursuit of Parenthood required sacrifices, but damn, an hour away? One way!

I came to this appointment... in the middle of a workday... three weeks after the results of my last blood test... and paid my co-pay... just to be told that I was being referred elsewhere. Especially right when tax season was starting at my new firm was picking up. This couldn't have been done via a phone call?

Seriously?

"Okay," I said. Ready to get out of there. I grabbed my purse and placed it on my lap. "Okay."

As she waxed poetic about how great McBride and her clinic were, I zoned out and worried about the time it would take to schedule this next appointment. I made myself focus again when I heard, "do you have any further questions for me?"

"Nope. I'm all set." And I wondered if that was true.

"Okay, just stop by registration before you leave to confirm your billing information and sign some paperwork saying that you approve of the referral and sharing of medical information, and we'll get that right over to them."

She stood up and opened the door. "I really hope Dr. McBride can give you some appropriate answers, and best of luck to you and Josh. She truly is great with patients experiencing infertility. I'm hoping that she'll be able to help you, too." She turned and headed out the door.

As I followed, I rooted in my purse for my phone and dialed up Josh. Time for another update.

Eleven

THE NEXT TWO MONTHS flew by in a blur. The earliest appointment we could get with Dr. McBride was for March 29, but for the first time in almost two years, the wait wasn't dragging at me. I was too busy to be counting the minutes.

It was the first tax season at my new accounting firm, and I was starting to regret asking to be salary rather than hourly. As a senior accountant there, I was not only preparing returns, but also reviewing some, and the responsibility was exhausting. On top of tax prep, I was also helping convert various clients to online accounting systems and, on other occasions, deal with IRS notices. Starting mid-to-late January, I was putting in fifty-five to sixty hours a week, and as the first March 15 deadline approached, I averaged around seventy-five hours per week. The week of the deadline, I hit eighty hours. Safe to say, I was toast.

But on the plus side, we saved a bunch of money on OPKs because I certainly didn't have the brainpower to try timing any coitus (as Dr. Sheldon Cooper would say).

While my coworkers were raking in that overtime dough, I was cursing myself for not thinking ahead, especially when Josh and I received a thick, little envelope from the clinic one day after work.

That special little package had not one, not two, but at least ten different billing statements enclosed. All the appointments where I requested to be billed later after things went through insurance... Well, the time had come to pay the piper. And apparently, the billing department fell a little behind and sent them all together to save on postage. The sticker shock was alarming.

As a rule, I had fairly good insurance. But that only takes you so far when you have a high deductible and out-of-pocket max. I recognized that it could have been worse - my plan partially covered infertility diagnosis. So even though I had to pay up to my out-of-pocket max for all the testing, at least it had a maximum amount, so it capped out. The negative is that it all happened right before the new year, which resulted in an out-of-pocket reset. So now I had to hit that metric all over again in the current year.

Not only was I cringing at the amounts that I was paying via credit card, but now I was wondering, 'if I can't afford to conceive a baby, do I have any business *having* a baby?' A throwback echoing from the horrid lady from our honeymoon ATV ride. Obviously, that was slightly dramatic, as Josh and I were financially sound enough that we could pay those invoices, given that we had delayed (partially not on purpose, thanks to infertility) getting pregnant. So, we had money saved up. Of course, that money was supposed to go to savings accounts, 529 plans, and baby gear–but alas, once again, you make plans, and God laughs.

Boom.

Curveball.

Life was certainly changing my perspective on things.

Snotty comments from people, parking tickets, leaky faucet, broken pipe, car accident, car broke down, etc. All of it could be worse. Infertility was changing my view of the universe. It was now viewed in terms of "well, it's not infertility."

There was this crippling doubt that I might never have a child of my own, and it was near paralyzing. I used to dream that we'd have a child that would be a unique blend of Josh and me. I used to dream that I would see my interesting eyes, which I inherited from my dad, passed down to my own kid. Now, fear had evolved and mutated my dreams for the future. Rather than assuming 'when' I had a baby, now it had changed to an 'if.' That fear was genuine. The longer it took for us to get pregnant, the more I gave up on those dreams and started thinking of alternatives. Maybe adoption would be the way to go. Or back onto the foster train.

We decided that donor eggs or sperm weren't options for us. Josh had mentioned that he'd prefer not to do the whole donated sperm thing if it came down to that. He said that if it was going to be biologically our child, then he wanted it to be both of our DNA, not just one. I was okay with that. We were in this together. It would either be both of our DNA or neither.

During the wait for our initial consult with Dr. McBride, Josh received a referral to a urologist at our clinic that basically told him he "didn't do" male reproductive issues and focused on the geriatric side of things. It was a dud of an appointment and didn't get us any closer to finding out if Josh's low count was genetic, hormonal, or a physical issue. As he was the only urologist in our hospital, we hoped that McBride's team would have someone better that could work with us.

As we sat in the waiting room, I felt a wave of relief that we were finally at the point where we could attend appointments together. More or less, we had pinpointed the issue. We didn't know what was causing the problem entirely, but we knew (or thought we knew) where the infertility stemmed from.

But what if it wasn't? What if there was something else going on too? We still never figured out the cause of my high prolactin levels and why my ovulation predictor tests were sometimes wonky...

What if there was still an issue with me, and we just missed it?

The drive over to the new clinic wasn't too bad. Getting insurance to approve the cross-border referral to a Vermont hospital when I was a New Hampshire resident had been tricky. As Josh perused the sports illustrated magazines on the side table, I inspected the wall art. In the waiting room, there were variations of slightly what some might consider pornographic flowers. Never having realized that certain flowers look so much like female anatomy. I was wondering at this revelation when they called our names and escorted us back to an exam room.

As this was the initial consult, no exam needed to be performed, and I think it just acted as an introduction of sorts. As I sat down next to

Josh to wait for Dr. McBride, I focused on the lesbian couple featured on the wall in front of me with their two adorable children. It looked like a photograph and not a stock photo. So maybe they were prior patients? I forced my mind to focus on that rather than obsessing over what was about to happen.

As Dr. McBride entered the room, Josh grabbed my hand and squeezed it with reassurance. "Ashley. Josh. I'm Dr. McBride. It's a pleasure to meet you."

As we exchanged introductions, I warmed up to yet another new doctor. She seemed very kind and knowledgeable. However, she gave me pause when she said, "Now, I know that you already did a lot of testing with Dr. Bradlee, but I'd like to redo some of her tests just to make sure we have the latest data. So, I want to put in an order to have your blood redrawn and another semen analysis done. Ashley, you can either use the lab here or back at your normal clinic. Josh... I wasn't thrilled with the results and analysis of your two prior semen analyses. I'd like you to redo yours, but I'd like you to redo it with a urologist that I work with frequently out of Massachusetts. He'll be a bit of a drive for you, but he's incredibly knowledgeable and skilled. I think he'll be able to interpret your results much more accurately."

I could tell that Josh was just going to leave it at that, so I jumped in. "Is there a chance that something could be wrong with Josh? Something we need to worry about?" I paused a beat. "Beyond infertility, I mean."

"You never really know with these sorts of things. It's one of those situations where it could be several reasons causing his unusual count. The Urologist will find out for sure. But with your family history being unremarkable," she was now looking at Josh directly, "I'm not overly concerned that this is stemming from something serious."

I breathed a metaphorical sigh of relief and looked over at Josh. He continued to look completely unbothered by this news. He's not one to borrow tomorrow's problems today, so I shouldn't have been surprised by his lack of concern.

He jumped in to clarify. "So, this urologist is based out of Boston?"

"Correct. Or should I say, just outside of Boston, but close enough to count. He comes up to the New Hampshire / Vermont area periodically, but that's usually only every couple of months. He won't be back up for another month or two because he was just here a week ago. When you call his office to schedule an appointment, they'll let you decide if you want to wait for him to come up here or if you'd prefer to see him sooner and go down there."

"Down there!" I rushed to say.

She smiled at my outburst and said, "I figured as much. Most couples that have waited as long as you two have are more than ready for the waiting game to be over."

"You can say that again," Josh muttered while squeezing my knee in solidarity.

"Call him when you are ready and set something up." She handed Josh the Urologist's card. "I'll put in the order for your bloodwork today as well, and we'll get things moving. Provided there is nothing we can do for Josh's count situation, we're likely looking at IVF, not IUI, as the semen count just isn't there to gamble on an IUI's success rate. Regardless, we'll know more after the follow-up tests and visits." With that parting shot, she shook our hands, said a quick goodbye, and left.

As Josh gave me his hand, I pulled myself up from my chair with a smile, squeezed his hand, and didn't let go. We left the clinic, and Josh indulgently let me prattle on about when and where I should schedule my blood tests. On the one hand, my normal lab was much closer. However, on the other, if we used McBride's lab, she could get the results sooner. My impatient side was leaning toward that option. I asked his opinion and was greeted with silence. Josh's face was buried in his phone, and he didn't look up once as we walked. We arrived at the car. I went to the driver's side and folded in as Josh did the same on the passenger side. I was felt slighted by his inattention and got snappish.

"I'm sorry, am I interrupting?" I facetiously inquired.

He frowned at me, mild disappointment in his expression. He looked back down at his phone, did something on the screen, and then put it to his ear.

"Hello, this is Josh... Yes, I did just send that email. Like I said, I would like the first available appointment, my work schedule is fairly flexible."

Whoopsie. I should have reeled in my 'bitch.'

"My bad. Sorry," I mouthed to him.

He waved a hand nonchalantly and continued speaking. "Yes... that would be fine. No, I used my phone earlier to see how best to get there. I don't need directions. That works. Umm," he paused. "Maybe two hours, depending on the time of day and traffic. Great, see you then."

He put his phone down and raised his eyebrows at me. Properly feeling chastised for being bitchy, I squeaked out, "sorry?" In my best meek, don't-be-mad-at-me voice. He wasn't buying it, so he rolled his eyes, sat back in his seat, and put on his seatbelt.

My excitement got the better of me. "So, you have an appointment already?" I was bursting with anxious energy. It wasn't even my appointment, but progress was progress.

He reached over, tugged my ponytail, and smiled. Apparently, no hard feelings. "Yup, your favorite day. April 15."

"But that's a Saturday this year?"

"I guess his office makes appointments on Saturdays. It's two weeks from now, I was hoping for sooner, but the rational part of me was impressed they squeezed me in with two weeks' notice. I'm not complaining."

We briefly discussed our next steps but moved on quickly to other topics. One thing about traveling with Josh, no matter whether it was a twenty-minute car ride or twenty hours, we never lacked for conversation. He was my best friend, and no topic was too weird for us to discuss. From periods to powerlifting, work to sports, we had a conversation-heavy relationship, and it always made road trips, no matter the length, enjoyable.

We talked about how I had been asked back to the softball team for this upcoming spring and summer and was eager to see my teammates again. Also, a local men's rugby team invited Josh to play for them, so he was debating on that. He had never played rugby before and was concerned that it would interfere with his powerlifting goals. He had just competed in his first state meet a couple of months prior and placed first in his weight class. Because it was his entrance into the powerlifting scene, and because he did so well, he was drug tested right after his meet. Watching him walk back to the bathroom with a meet official escorting him so they could watch him pee in a cup was hilarious. Because the USAPL (USA Powerlifting) is drug-free, they take their testing seriously. Obviously, he passed.

It was a little extra funny because each doctor we had seen so far had asked the same questions about whether Josh had ever taken steroids or testosterone boosters, given his weightlifting hobby. We assured them it wasn't the case and that he was clean. I had worries about his caffeine intake based on some of the research I had seen online, but every doctor we spoke to assured us that caffeine wasn't a likely infertility driver.

As I drove, I also vented about tax season and how overwhelmed I felt. I was so tired and mentally stressed. The hours were killing me. Combine work-related stress with the infertility-related stress, and I felt like I was strung tighter than a bowstring. With Dr. McBride's parting shot about possibly needing to do IVF, now I might be adding financial stress to my list. Each appointment and test was eating away at our nest egg. We were now several thousand dollars down, and with a new deductible for the current year, and again, possibly IVF in our future, I thought that we needed to re-evaluate our budget.

Our budget.

happy mental sigh

I loved that thing.

Josh and I updated it and revised it every couple of months. Every pay change, every bonus, every coaching paycheck, every contribution to our retirement accounts. I had a section broken out for monthly expenses so we could see our cash flow. I also had a section for once-a-year expenses (oil, IRA funding, house projects, Christmas presents, etc.). I wasn't as neurotic as my new boss (who had his expenses down to the penny in QuickBooks Online), but Josh and I had a pretty good system going. We had a section budgeted out for medical and a category called 'baby.' I'd kept a tally of the bills as they came in, and we were already nearly at our budget. We could start taking away from some of our other budgeted categories, and we had retirement and emergency savings, but obviously, those were supposed to be our last resort.

I flicked on my blinker to merge onto the highway and said to Josh, "Should we look into starting a GoFundMe for some of these expenses?"

He looked at me like I was crazy. "No!" He blurted out. "It's not anyone else's responsibility to pay for us to have a kid!" He looked aghast.

"People obviously wouldn't *have* to donate. They could just donate if they wanted to." I mumbled.

"Dude. No." He stressed. "It's no one's business. I can't believe you'd be willing to accept handouts for that. That's not like you at all."

"I know." I sighed. "I'm just trying to think of options if we run out of money."

"We're not there yet."

"I know," I emphasized.

"So, let's not worry about it yet."

"But by then, it might be too late. We should try to plan, so we have things in place, so things don't have to stall." I tried to rationalize.

"Ash," he groaned. "We don't know if it will get to that point. Do you really want to go from no one knowing about all this to *everyone* knowing? I mean, really? Just the other day, you were at lunch with what's-her-name, and she was talking about how her sister-in-law was doing IVF for the fourth time. Then went off about how sometimes there are *reasons* why sperm can't fertilize an egg and how basic biology was trying to tell them that a child between them isn't biologically sanctioned. She went on and on to you about how science meddles in that and how it's unnatural. Then she dragged religion into it and started on Catholicism and how they don't approve of IVF and how her sister-in-law is going against nature and God by doing IVF. It was a train wreck. You came home that night in tears! Do you really want to open yourself up to more of that?"

"To be fair, she didn't know we were going through something similar..." I said meekly, semi-trying to defend her. But yeah, that conversation had been particularly painful to get through without saying something I'd later regret.

"But doing a GoFundMe opens you up to situations like that."

I passed a car on the left and merged back into the right lane. I glanced quickly at Josh. "I don't super love the idea. It was just a thought."

"You were *so* upset that night, Ash." He repeated.

"It just was a lot to handle. And it was 3/15 week. Emotions were running high."

"If you say so."

"So." Out of the corner of my eye, I saw him look at me and smile before facing forward again.

And that was that. I let it lie for now, but I'd monitor our budget and creeping expenses and bring up the subject again when I needed to. But he was right; I had enough on my mind for the time being. Maybe I should just focus on the next few steps before putting the cart before the horse.

We moved on and enjoyed our hour-long ride home. After arriving home, I caught up on some tax returns from the home office. Josh worked out downstairs, and then we connected again for a late dinner. We said our goodnights, and I worked until twelve-thirty, trying to finish up a return. I was also late-night texting my friend Jamie with our results and commiserating with her about their delay in getting pregnant. She was feeling the burn of missed months as well. I finished up the return, signed off, and as I was sliding into bed when my phone chimed with a text. I thought it was Jamie again, but it was another friend from high school.

In the body of the text message was a chubby, whopper of a newborn baby boy that looked like he ate entire chickens for breakfast. Proud mom and dad were cuddling him close.

I looked at her exhausted face and her husband's slightly queasy-looking smile and then back to the little chunk in their arms. I shot back my congratulations texts and put my phone away. I curled deep into Josh, shoving my icy toes between his thighs. His body didn't even move from the chill. I threw my arm around him and buried closer. I tried to calm my mind, but I kept seeing the joy on their faces. They were on Cloud Nine. *Walking on sunshine.* They were living the dream. And we might never have that. *Will I ever become a mother?* The doctor's comments from today came rushing back. We might have to do IVF. IVF would give us a 30-40% chance, if lucky.

The shaking started in my lower jaw at first. The quivering was unexpected but fierce. My breath came a little quicker and was slowly getting louder than our fan, which was set on low. As the emotion gained traction, my breaths became much smaller and choppier. My eyes were burning, so I squeezed them tighter. My nose ran, and my ears were ringing. Within a minute, I was full-on shaking everywhere and clinging to Josh with all my might as I heaved in breath after breath.

As I tried harder to pull in more air to calm down and regulate myself, my throat just became more and more irritated. Before I knew it, I started emitting a squawking sound on each inhale as I scraped and dragged air into my lungs. The asthma attack woke Josh with a start. "What the fuck?" He half mumbled, half queried. He rolled over to look at me and shot up in bed. "Jesus Ash. Sit up, sit up. Arms above your head. Deep breaths, deep breaths." He started taking deep breaths to trick my body into trying to breathe with him, but I was too far gone.

My vision turned narrow; everything was in a tunnel.

All I could hear were my own labored breaths.

I was sweating and cold at the same time.

I couldn't stop shaking.

My arms felt weak as I tried to lift them over my head to open my lungs.

But I was just so tired.

When my body processed it wasn't getting nearly enough oxygen, adrenaline started coursing and triggered my panic reflex. So the laboring just intensified as my body fought harder for each breath... Josh's face popped into view. "Where's your inhaler, Ash? Where is it?"

I tried to answer, but couldn't, unable to get enough air to form words. I scraped in another breath, dropping my hands from above my head and tugging at the skin of the base of my throat. It felt too tight, too narrow. Maybe if I pulled at my skin hard enough, it would open up my airway. It was like breathing through a swizzle stick. Even though a part of me knew it wouldn't help (I developed asthma as a kid, so had been around the block a time or two), I still weakly pulled at my neck. Rational thinking has no place during an asthma attack.

I saw Josh take off out of the room and absently wondered what would happen if I passed out. Would my body still struggle to breathe? Or would the panic cease, and my body would just regulate itself? Inhalers aren't immediate. They take ten to fifteen minutes to really kick in. Even if he got the inhaler, it would do no use until I could breathe enough to take it. At this rate, I wouldn't have enough breath regulation to inhale, hold, and exhale. I'd pass out.

I needed to get ahold of myself.

I just... couldn't. I couldn't slow my panicked breaths down.

Josh ran back into the room and came next to me on the bed, looking down to where my hands were pulling at my throat while he held the inhaler up to my lips. I tried to move my head away, knowing it wouldn't help. The first step needed to be of my own control, but he put it back to my mouth. I pulled my hand away from my neck and grabbed the inhaler. I tried to inhale slowly and pushed the canister down to disburse the albuterol, but my breath was too shallow and too quick. I didn't have a spacer for my inhaler, and because I was shaking so much, I sprayed most of the medicine on my teeth and lips. I tried taking another breath before trying the inhaler again. My airway closed on me. Looking at Josh in terror, I grabbed at my throat. He grabbed his phone from the nightstand and asked urgently, "Do I call someone?"

My airway stopped seizing long enough for me to drag in another short and noisy breath. The exhale was quick and not nearly as loud. I tried sucking in another breath. The same thing happened. Airway closed. A choking noise poured from my throat. My hand went from my throat to Josh, where I grabbed his arm hard. He leaned into me and started taking deep, slow breaths. He gave me a choice. "Either get this regulated on your own, or I'm calling 911. Deep breaths with me. In and out. In and out. Slow and deep. That's it."

He channeled his inner Zen and pushed it at me with his eyes. He learned years ago not to touch me during asthma attacks. Hands-on my back or head and rubbing my back were all not good for me. He could let me hold on to his hands, but I couldn't be restrained. Having someone else touch me during an asthma attack felt too hot. Too heavy. Too suffocating.

As he completed his slow, controlled breaths in front of me, I focused my scattered thoughts on nothing but trying to mimic his breathing. My body wouldn't stop shaking, and tears drenched my cheeks. I could feel the sweat drip from my hairline onto my face, quickly joining the highway of tears down my face and chin. I'd have a few controlled breaths and then an uneven, gasping one, but then a couple more good breaths. It wasn't perfect, but it was enough to get down some albuterol into my lungs. I took four puffs over the course of a few minutes - not exactly as prescribed, but I just wanted it in my system. After a couple minutes, I had more regulated breaths than choking ones. I let my death grip on Josh's forearm go, but he didn't move. He continued to look at me and modeled deep breathing. He lifted a hand and gently swiped away some tears from the apple of my cheek and smiled softly as he took another long, slow inhale. I mimicked him, though mine was much shakier. My hands were vibrating from adrenaline, nerves, and maybe a bit from the albuterol hitting my system. After asthma attacks, I was always shaky and as weak as a kitten.

"I'll go get some water?" Josh queried softly.

I nodded.

He slipped out of the room and returned quickly with water from the tap. I grabbed it on unsteady fingers and brought it to my lips, nearly sloshing some out of the side. I anchored the glass against my chin as I tipped it up, but my whole body was quivering, so it didn't stabilize it all that much. As I took a sip, I felt some dribble onto my chin. Even with the tiny sip, it triggered a mini coughing fit. My lungs and airway felt like they were on fire and sore. My nose was still running, and I looked around for the tissue box. Josh saw where I was looking and lurched over to grab it for me. I smiled my thanks and grabbed one, trying to settle my breathing enough to use the tissue. By the time I was done blowing, folding over, blowing, folding over, the tissue was soaked. Yuck.

Josh waited until I was done and then queried softly, "what brought that on?"

"I just... I... I... I just," I sniffed, "I got overwhelmed. Tax season and work and the baby stuff and money stuff and the appointment today. It just all hit me, and I was suffocating. I'm so tired—both literally and figuratively.

I'm getting no sleep because of tax season hours, but that will be over soon. Just a couple more weeks." I coughed quietly. "And I shouldn't complain about lack of sleep. Newborns give their parents even fewer hours of sleep, right?" Josh looked unimpressed. I continued. "I just," I paused. "What if we run out of money before we can finish IVF? Do we cash out our retirement funds? What if IVF doesn't work for us? What do we do then? Adoption is as expensive, if not more so. Fostering is great and all, but I don't want to fall in love and then have them taken away. And maybe, maybe Wendy was right. Maybe there's a reason we can't get pregnant. Maybe we're not supposed to?" I trailed off, wispy and hoarse from my attack.

"Don't be finding those Catholic roots on me now." Josh fake warned, and I felt my lips turn up slightly, as he intended. "There's no master plan that says that we're not supposed to have kids. Don't take that on. If you want to listen to the zealots that say if you were meant to get pregnant, then God would get you pregnant... then you have to try the shoe on the other foot as well. Maybe, if God didn't want you to get pregnant, maybe he wouldn't let IVF be a thing. But, all that's prescribing to the ideology that God has a plan for everyone rather than letting everyone have autonomy over his own life. And you know, dear, I'm not even sure I believe in God, so I'm not the best person to talk to about it." He smiled sheepishly. "But how did I do? Calm your fears?"

I smiled at him again. "You did fine, champ," I reassured him weakly. "I'm fine now. It all just overwhelmed me for a minute. Just a thought that got a little out of control, and spiraled. I'm back to regularly scheduled programming. No more freak-outs. For now..." I hastened to add. "I reserve the right to freak out again later." He leaned forward and kissed my sweaty and clammy forehead.

"You wouldn't be you if you didn't." He smiled back at me. "Do you want to talk about it some more?"

"No, I just want to sleep."

"You're still shaking." He noted.

"Yeah, I will be for a while. It's the albuterol, plus it's always worse after an attack. Now I'm exhausted, more than I already was, so let's just go back to bed."

Josh scrutinized my face, found what he was looking for, and nodded. He pulled back the covers for me and slid beside me, pulling me close.

"Ash, I promise you, no matter what, no matter what happens, I promise you, I *promise* you, we will become parents. There's no doubt in my mind. We will make sure that happens. It might take a bit, but we'll get there. Promise."

I felt his vow sink deep into me, and I realized with tired surprise that he was right. It might take a bit, but we were meant to be parents. We had too much love to give and too much to offer to help shape the world. We would do this. Like Josh said, one way or another, we would find a way. *Little did I know that this joint decision became the foundation of my drive, rooted deeply in my spirit... Keeping me afloat and breathing.*

Twelve

"How's the baby making going?" Alaina asked while sipping her lemonade.

I hesitated for a second and then gave her the truth. "It's disheartening. I've said it before, and I'm sure I'll say it again, but it's frustrating that my body can't do the one thing that it's supposed to do. It's also weird to look back at our high school years and how all the teachers convinced us that we'd end up pregnant the first time we had unprotected sex. And here I am. Not pregnant. After years. It's just... ironic?"

She nodded in solidarity. "It's depressing to see how easily some people get pregnant and don't deserve it and then watch how hard you and Josh have tried."

"It is what it is." I shrugged again, took a sip of my water, and looked around the restaurant's outside patio.

The waitress walked quickly by our table, an older couple trailing her slowly. The lady's purse bumped into the back of my chair, causing my purse to fall to the ground. I leaned over to pick it up, and when I sat back up, I saw Alaina scrolling on her phone.

She tucked her blonde hair behind her ear, winced slightly, and took a deep breath. "So, I know you've probably tried all of this, but we haven't really discussed it. I want to at least chat about it first in case you didn't read about any of these ideas."

I braced myself. This sounded... ominous.

I took a bite of my sandwich. After I swallowed, I affirmed out, "shoot."

"Okay." She started. "You charted your cycle every month and pinpointed your ovulation times?"

"Roger that."

"Did you guys have sex every day leading up to and during the ovulation window, or did you do it every couple of days? Depending on who you listen to can affect your chances. Some people say one way is more effective than the other."

"Yes, dear." I agreed, mock placatingly. "We tried it both ways. We had lots of data points to choose from during the last two years. However, it got to where Josh was struggling to even get into the mood and have sex with me at all during the ovulation window because there was so much pressure. I had to stop telling him for a while because otherwise, his erection would die quicker than a snowflake on a summer day in Florida." I lowered my voice at the end. Talking about Josh's performance issues felt like a betrayal of him, so I left it at that. But it was 100% the truth. After a certain point, it was like he physically couldn't get his body to have sex with me with all the pressure. And showing any frustration with that impotence was NOT the way to improve the mood.

She nodded brusquely, took another sip, and kept going down her list–that was apparently compiled on her phone.

"After sex, did you lay with your feet in the air for ten to fifteen minutes to help the sperm reach the motherland?"

I choked out a laugh, looked around, and shook my head in disbelief. Only Alaina would discuss this at lunchtime in a public place. Thankfully, we didn't have many people around us.

"Again, yes. I tried that as well." This was a little embarrassing. But she was a nurse, so she had probably heard it all. The hope was that gravity would help the little buggers join the superhighway into my cervix and find an egg. It didn't seem to work for us. *Obviously*.

"Did you try being in certain positions during the male climax? Also, did you ensure that you were achieving your end of the things?" She winked conspiratorially at me, and I smiled. "Some sites I was reading said that the aftershocks and pulses post-orgasm can help migrate the sperm to where they need to go."

I took another healthy bite of my sandwich and hummed in agreement.

I was in a good headspace today. No depression cloud looming over me. Otherwise, these questions would be much rougher for me to handle. I was viewing the entire scenario as humorous rather than depressing, contrary to how I was viewing most fertility conversations lately.

"Okay, so that's out." She scrolled some more on her phone, absently taking a bite of her French fry. "Did you use lubrication? Some say it can help; others say it damages the sperm. So there's mixed information out there."

"We also tried using Pre-seed lubrication to help the sperm shoot right up to the motherland." I sighed. "Trust me, Alaina. There's mixed information about everything. What one person calls 'red,' another will call 'orange.' There are very few answers. I've even drank Fertili-Tea and tried using essential oils. I've tried it all." I was actually very impressed with myself and how calm and mature I sounded, rather than how frustrated and hopeless I really felt.

"Okay, okay. I'll stop now. Thanks for humoring me. I just wanted to mention some of the things I was reading about." She reached over and patted my hand twice. "So now that we got that out of the way.

Now for the fun parts." She pulled her hand back and started rummaging around in her purse. She pulled out a couple of pink... rocks...Rocks?

"These are rose quartz stones. My aunt said that if you put them on your pillow at night, the energy from the stones can help you get pregnant. She gave them to me a year ago, and now I have a baby. It might be nothing. It might be something. She told me to be careful putting them too close together, though, because she said that it increases the likelihood of twins. So, if you're okay with that... might as well give these try."

I blinked at her. I opened my mouth to say something, I wasn't sure what, then closed it again. After opening my mouth again, I paused before making a sound. She had a sheepish look on her face.

"What did you do with my friend, and who are you?" I choked out. And then laughed outright; she joined in, though hers had an undercurrent of embarrassment, and her cheeks pinkened.

"I know! I know it's not like me! But if you've tried everything else, you might as well try this too! Who knows if it will work?"

I started laughing harder.

"Well, if you're going to be a bitch about it," she groused as she reached over to return the stones to her purse - her nose in the air. "Hmmm, after that, maybe you can find your own rose quartz crystals."

I sobered up quickly and shot my hand out to cover the stones. "Nope! I'll try them! It doesn't hurt. I can put them right next to the essential oils that my mom bought me. Apparently, they also can increase fertility."

"I'm sorry I laughed." I fake apologized. "You've just never bought into hocus-pocus stuff before, so I was shocked!"

"Yeah, yeah," she waved me off. Not buying my apology for a minute. "Well, after that reception, it makes me not want to give you my other present, but luckily for you, I'm a good friend and won't hold your poor behavior against you." She sniffed haughtily and looked in her purse again.

This time, she came out with a bottle of cold medicine. The bottle was already half empty, and I could feel my cheeks lift again, but I held in any bubbling laughs that might try to escape.

"It's cold syrup. It loosens up the mucus in your body. It is great for colds, but there's a theory that it will also make your vaginal secretions less viscous and waterier, so the sperm have an easier path to travel. I took a little each day, and boom, pregnant. Maybe it will work for you?" She looked a little pink around the ears again. I swallowed any smart-ass retort, took the bottle, and looked at her earnest expression.

"Thank you, Lain. I appreciate you looking into all this for me and trying to help. And you're right, and it doesn't hurt."

"You were going through this solo for so long. And I know it wasn't easy watching me get married, get pregnant, and have a baby all in the same time span that you were desperately trying for yourself. I just wanted to make sure you knew the door was always open to talk about stuff. And if you don't want to talk, then that's cool too."

"I know," I smiled softly. "Thank you." I felt like a rotten friend for being so envious of her happiness for the last two years. I'd do better, I vowed to myself.

"Oh! Another thing, have you guys talked about getting on an adoption waitlist at all while you wait? Just in case? Your mom's family was adopted, right?"

"Yeah, they all were. All from different families. Josh's family has a bunch of adopted kids, too."

"Have you guys discussed that as an option?"

I nodded. "Yeah, we have—multiple times. I even spoke with an adoption specialist a month or two ago. She squashed any ideas pretty quick."

Her brows puckered. "What do you mean?"

Before jumping in, I took a quick bite and washed it down with my water. "She said that they won't even work with us until we've officially stopped trying to have a baby of our own. She said that acknowledging that we're not having our own biological child will usually result in a type of depression and grieving process. Essentially, the acceptance of giving up on our preconceived notions about what our family will look like and the grief that we will never see in our eyes or mouth or chin in our children's faces can basically be a grieving process. So they require families to go through that and heal before even starting the adoption process. They don't want us to view adoption as a backup method of achieving a kid and then back out once we get pregnant."

"Damn." She whistled low. "That's harsh."

"Totally." I sighed. "But I can see why. From all my research and the discussions that Josh and I have had, there's so much to even consider. Age, siblings, gender, ethnicity, open adoption, special needs, on and on. It's intense."

"I don't know if I could do an open adoption," she murmured.

"Same." I retorted. But who knew? Maybe if that was our only option, I'd be jumping at the chance. I've been finding more and more that my expectations of myself and my perfectly planned out life were *very* subject to change. "Who knows?" I added on, echoing my thoughts. "Who knows."

Thirteen

I WAS ENJOYING A nice round of end-of-tax-season celebratory golf when Josh called with an update on his appointment with the Urologist.

"Hey there, what are you up to?"

"My parents took me golfing. We're only on the second hole, but I think I fixed my slice from last year!" I said optimistically. And probably incorrectly. "How did the appointment go?"

"Do you have time to talk, or do you want to call me later?"

"Nah, I just teed off, so I'm all set. If nothing else, I can just sit in the cart and chat and just pick up my ball. It's not like I'm playing for stakes."

"Alrighty then. So you know how I texted you when I got there, and I told you they were running late?"

"Yes."

"Well, they were running *really* late. They were forty-five minutes late by the time the doctor came to talk to me."

"Jeez! And on Saturday, no less!"

"Yeah, there weren't even that many people in the waiting room, so I don't know what was happening. But after waiting for fifteen minutes or so, I took a nap."

I cut in, "Naturally."

"Yeah, yeah, I know." I could hear his smile. "Anyway, so I took a nap, and then I got woken up by the receptionist, which was great, so I geared myself up to talk to the doc, but she woke me up just to escort me to a room. She said I was snoring and looked tired, so she said I could nap in one of the assessment rooms."

"Did you?"

"Did I what?"

"Nap in the assessment room?"

"No way. My adrenaline had already rallied me from being woken up. So I just sat there and twiddled my thumbs. Kind of a bummer she woke me."

"What a bitch." I said sarcastically.

"My thoughts exactly." I could hear him smile.

"So what next?"

"So the doc came in and told me that my semen morphology was abnormal. But we knew that. What the Urologist back home didn't say to us was that most men have abnormal semen results. Of one variety or another. Or at least, that's what this doc said. He said my count was abysmally low. But on the plus side, I was producing sperm at least, just not very much. That could be attributed to several things: a blockage in my urethra, a genetic issue, or a blockage elsewhere in the gonadal region."

"Okay, we kind of already knew this, right?"

"Right," he agreed. "So basically, he wants a semen analysis done at his clinic because he had an issue with the prior interpretations, and then wants a follow-up where he can run some tests himself."

I rolled my eyes. "Another semen analysis?"

"Hey, we're at the end of the line on narrowing down the problem. If I have to splooge in a cup to get this done, no problem. Plus, this time, I'm not likely to run into my father-in-law... Unless... Does your father have a urologist he sees near Boston?"

"Not that I know of!" I chuckled. "Want me to ask? He's right next to me?"

"Nah, I'm good," he laughed back.

"Okay, so do you have the next steps already scheduled on the family calendar?"

"Yup, I'll do that before I leave here and head home. I'll be back in about two hours. Want me to pick up dinner when I come through town?"

"Sure. My usual at Panera, please?"

"You got it, babe. See you when I get home."

"Love you."

"Bye."

"How did it go?" My mom rushed to ask.

"Still no answers, but we're getting closer."

As I listened to my mom lament the slow process and question why we didn't have answers yet, I felt like this was possibly the definition of irony. I was never clear on the definition: deciding whether something was ironic or coincidental or just simply humorous. As she ranted about how it was ridiculous that the doctors couldn't figure this out, I thought how funny it was that these were usually *my* lines. And now, here I was, reassuring her it was getting done. We were doing the best we could to stop fretting, to stop researching all the way things could go wrong or be wrong. Now that I was playing his role, I understood Josh a bit more. I made a tentative vow to myself to stop harping on all the way things could go south during this process. I was proud of my self-awareness but then went down the rabbit hole of wondering if I was truly self-aware and if I was patting myself on the back for it. And the mental onslaught continued.

I finished up the round of golf with my parents and headed home. After showering and getting dressed in my coziest clothes, I sat down at my computer and started researching the kinds of tests my husband could have on his next visit. My gut clenched as I read more and more. I started to sweat and cringe. Dear lord. That can't be right. My stomach felt queasy. So far in this process, he had definitely come out ahead - his tests were much less traumatic than mine. I thought this test might make us even. But I caught myself. I assumed this test was going to happen. Didn't I make a vow to myself earlier this afternoon to not go down the negative rabbit hole? Maybe this wasn't even the test that the Urologist was going to run.

"Ash, I'm home!" I heard a call from the kitchen.

"Hi dear, quick question!" I heard rustling brown paper bags as I made my way into the kitchen. Josh was laying out our romantic feast for two. He gave me a quick kiss and went to grab utensils from our drawer.

"Sure, what's up?" He asked.

"What was the test the Urologist wanted to run in a couple of weeks?"

"He wanted to do some ultrasounds and cyto-something. Why?" He moved to open his salad with chicken and sat down at the barstool.

"A cystoscopy?"

"Yeah! How'd you know?" He shoved a sizeable chunk into his mouth and started chewing. "Oh," he murmured.

"Yeah, I researched it."

"I'm putting that on your tombstone. That, and 'where's my phone?'"

I did say both of those quite a bit. The darn phone kept growing legs and moving on me. All the time.

"So, do you want to know what I found?"

"Nope."

"You don't want to hear what it is?" I pushed. "Not even a hint?"

"Nope, don't tell me."

"But- "

"Nope, not a word, Ash. I don't want to know."

"Oh, alright," I grumbled. "But you might regret this."

"Maybe, but I'm fine with taking that chance." He took another heaping bite. The iceberg lettuce crunched deliciously. I opened my mouth like a baby bird and leaned forward. He rolled his eyes, seared a crisp chunk of lettuce, and forked it into my mouth. Not bad.

As we sat and talked about my last day of tax season, I tried very hard to forget what I had learned during my research this evening. If he didn't want to know, I would not be the one to burst that happy bubble he was living in. I'd let him learn the hard way that sometimes being prepared is worth its weight in gold. I took a bite of warm gooey mac and cheese when a thought hit me, and I looked up at him quickly.

"Hey! Why are you so certain I'm going to die first?" I was mock insulted.

He just looked at his chicken and salad and then pointedly looked at my mac and cheese and chocolate brownie.

"Point taken," I said as I grinned cheekily at him and took another delicious bite.

I was paying some bills that had accumulated over tax season when Josh came and gave me a quick kiss goodbye. His second appointment was today, and he needed to get a jump on traffic.

"Can I take your car rather than my truck?"

"Sure. Safer and better on gas when driving toward Boston makes sense." I said absently as I totaled the numbers on my notepad in front of me.

"All right, I'm out of here. Call you after."

"Good luck!" I called as I heard the door shut.

I frowned at the computer screen and re-checked my math. I pulled out my phone's calculator and re-ran the numbers. Yup, our utility company hadn't cashed our check from a couple of months ago. I'd have to call them. Maybe I never dropped it off? Oh jeez, tax season brain strikes again!

I put a calendar appointment on my phone to call on Monday and ask about it because I found the only way I remembered stuff these days was to put it on the calendar with reminders and alerts. I wasn't always so scattered, but life had gotten complicated. How the mighty had fallen. I used to brag about my organizational skills, yet here I was, wondering if I forgot to pay our utility bill.

Out of curiosity, I started researching local IVF clinics and felt my stomach clench. There weren't many. Only a couple were within a two-hour drive. We could go north or south, that was it. At least the one up north was part of the same hospital chain as our local hospital. But the one down south had better success rates. Cost-wise, they were similar. Either way, we were looking at some four-to-five-digit bills. I dug deeper into the various aspects of IVF. In the past, I had always stopped once arriving at the IVF point. It seemed like such an unlikely outcome for two 'normal' people. But I guess that's what infertility is: it affects anyone and everyone, and no one is immune.

If nothing else, maybe I'd look back on this experience and say that it was a time of self-discovery. I had certainly *discovered* a lot. I had turned bitter, unhappy, and worrisome during the last two years. I was negative and overwhelmed, questioning and doubtful. In truth, I was a shade of the person I used to be. Playing with children and seeing family and friends used to bring me joy. I'd smile at kids in the grocery store and say 'ooos' over newborns. Now, I waved sadly at the kids and tried not to cry. Now, I smelled that newborn baby smell and just wanted to curl up in a ball and sob myself to sleep.

I was a shadow of the exuberant person I used to be. But, if nothing else, this process taught me I was also resilient and tough. Never compromising and willing to quit. Maybe I was harboring a secret optimism by continuing to get up every time life kicked me in the teeth. And I was well informed: resourceful and inquisitive. So even though life had me down, and I wasn't who I used to be, maybe this was just part of growing up. Maybe it was just finally 'my turn' to have something tough happen in my life. I had such a blessed life until now. If I wanted to go down a religious road, maybe this was my test.

Then again, maybe it was just life.

I spent the day finishing all the chores I had ignored during tax season. First, I had started with our bills, and then, hours later, I finished putting away old holiday decorations. Then, I spring-cleaned the house from top to bottom. To celebrate all my hard work, I soaked up some Vitamin D on the back patio while reading the latest Kristen Ashley book. When my phone started ringing, I placed it on speaker, shut off my Kindle Paperwhite, and reclined back. "Sock it to me, lovebug."

"So that was a fun visit, let me tell you."

I grinned.

"Well, I had about a forty-minute wait again, so at least they're consistent. That, or they expect everyone in Massachusetts to be a chronic late arrival, and they've budgeted that into their schedule."

"If I ever need to see a urologist, I'll go there. That sounds perfect to me. I'm always late... except for my period. That's never late."

"Only because you never know when you're going to freaking have it."

"It is curious that I can be that unpredictable and have my ovulation days so close to my period and have that not have any effect on our infertility.

They just kind of stopped looking at issues with me and just assumed it was you. Don't get me wrong. It definitely seems like it's mostly you. But it could be a bit me as well. Maybe I should ask them again if maybe it's both of us." I trailed off.

"You just want to be special like me." He teased.

"Oh, totally. I want that infertility card as well. Infertile people get all the best parking spots."

"I tell people you're with me for the money, but maybe I should amend and say you're with me for the infertility benefits."

"Yeah, that sounds much more likely."

"Okay, banter over. Moving on. So the ultrasound was first. But it wasn't one ultrasound. It was two. One was external on the testicles, and the other was transrectal. I wasn't expecting that one. Good thing I pooped this morning before leaving. Also, sidebar, that gel is seriously cold when it's used on your sack!"

I smiled as he intended and asked, "alright, so how did that go?"

"As unpleasant as that was at first, the good news is that I got used to the sensation after a couple of minutes. And because they sucked me into a TV show about an Australian vet in the waiting room, I didn't get to nap. I think you'd like him. He's very handsome and plays with animals all day; your kind of show!" I blinked at the quick subject change, but he brought it back just as quick. "Anyway, so I didn't get my nap, and I had to leave early this morning to get to my appointment in time, so I got a little drowsy in the ultrasound room. There was a fan going, and I was laying back, and it was dark..."

"You didn't!"

"I feel like I should say I'm not proud of myself, but I actually kind of am! As the technician was scanning away, I fell asleep. I could hear just how impressed he was with himself, and I shook my head, not that he could see me. "But then the doctor came in and *disturbed my slumber!*" He softly boomed in his best Aladdin voice, "the technician looked at him and said quietly, 'there are cysts *everywhere.*' So that was fun to hear."

"Are you serious?"

"Yeah, so that's not great to hear. Apparently, the pain that I have *down there* sometimes? I guess it's cysts rupturing or getting inflamed. Who knew!"

"Oh my God! Is that serious? Is there something we need to do? Can they fix it? Is there medication? Is that hereditary? I told you that you should have asked your doc about that years ago!" I shot the questions at him rapid-fire.

"He said that we could discuss surgery, but he didn't recommend it. One, because they could come back, and two, that there were also just so many of them it might do more harm than good."

"Oh my God, Josh. That's awful. Anything they can do for the pain, at least?"

"Nope."

"And they will not do anything about the cysts? Ever?"

"Nope again."

"Jeez, well, okay then."

"Pretty much. So anyway, the second ultrasound, as I said, was transrectal. Never in my life have I had something shoved up my butt, Ash. The technician was great, walking me through what was going on, so it wasn't super terrible or anything, but it wasn't exactly fun. She'd say, 'and now you're about to feel this sensation, et cetera, et cetera. Once the probe was way up there, I commented on how it was a little uncomfortable, to which she responded, 'you don't want stuff shoved up there too frequently, trust me.'"

"What does that mean?" I choked out a laugh.

"It means that she's a freak in the sheets and definitely takes it up the dooder."

I started laughing outright.

"So yeah, with those pearls of wisdom, I just bit my lip and endured it. Not too bad, though. But the Cystoscopy! Why didn't you warn me?" He half shouted.

I shot up indignantly, sputtering in outrage.

"Just kidding." He blurted. "They wanted to see if there was a blockage in my urethra, so they shoved a camera up my dick hole to look. Let me repeat. They shoved a camera up my dick hole." I cringed for him. "The first thing the doc did was stick a plastic syringe down there and insert some kind of gel into my dick hole. Dude, it was weird. I'm not sure if the gel was to 'fill me up' to make it easier to get in there or to act as an anesthetic."

"Or maybe both?" I suggested.

"Maybe." I could practically see him shrugging his shoulders in typical Josh-fashion. "Then he let it sit there for a bit and made awkward small talk while my dick was just hanging out. Then he pulled out a camera the length of your forearm and the diameter of a mechanical pencil. And then... in it went. It fucking sucked! The doctor was great. He tried his best to be calming, so he rambled a ton and it helped distract me. He gave me the grand tour of my urinary tract today. I could have died happy never going on that particular theme park ride. But the worst part was that I wanted to pee before driving home, and Ash... Ash, it was miserable. Oh my God. He warned me it might burn while peeing for a bit, and he was not wrong! Again, oh my god. I literally thought I was going to vomit while peeing. You know my pain tolerance. It takes a lot for me to feel that way. But oh my God. I started gagging. It hurt so bad. Plus, he said I might have blood in my urine, so I shouldn't be freaked. My eyes were squeezed so tight I didn't know if there was blood, but he said it would last a few days, so I guess I have more chances to see it. Lucky me."

"Eek, well, hopefully, the next place doesn't make you have to redo this test."

He gasped in horror. "Why would you even say that?"

"Well, it seems like every doctor we talk to doesn't like the previous doctor's tests and interpretations. Case in point: how many semen analyses have you done so far?"

"Yeah, no. I'm hoping that's not a thing I have to do again. Though, for a baby, I gotta do what I gotta do. You know?"

"Mmm," I agreed.

"So I sat down with the doc after and went over everything, and he assured me they were benign and not to worry. And he gave us the final decision that those caused my low sperm count. So there we have it. The smoking gun. The cause of all this drama and heartache. I have myself some cysts." He said the last like a Southern auctioneer. "I asked him if it was possible for us to conceive naturally, and he gave me a visible pause. So, I took a leaf out of your book and asked him if it was akin to Jim Carrey's chances in Dumb and Dumber."

"So you're saying there's a chance?"

"Yeah, he didn't get it, so I had to clarify. It killed the attempt at humor. Anyway, our chances are more like one in a million. Not really something we should hang our hats on. We have similar odds of winning the Lottery this week. But, the other good news is that we never have to worry about birth control ever again. Yay." He said the last half-heartedly, but tried to be positive, so I appreciated that. "I think it's similar to playing Russian Roulette... with one of those massive machine guns with chains and ammunition, but only one bullet is live. So it's possible, just not likely."

"Well, that's a bummer. Not about the no birth control piece, but the rest of it. I was hoping they'd find something that they could actually fix. But oh well, I guess. We have our answer finally."

"It's all on me, dear. I'm sorry." He breathed.

"Josh. No. It's not your fault. Just like you wouldn't blame me for a bum uterus. I don't hold this against you. We'll get through this. We'll be fine." Here I was, playing Josh's usual role and reassuring him for a change. Another personal growth moment for me.

"I guess just put it on our calendar for us to call McBride on Monday and set up a follow-up appointment. Before I left, they said that they'd pass along the results to her today so her office should know that we're coming back."

"IVF, here we come," I said, trepidation clear in my voice.

"IVF, here. We. Come." He echoed.

Fourteen

I WAS OBSESSIVELY CHECKING the clock on my computer screen and feeling nauseous. Today was the day that I wanted to officially communicate my fertility struggles to my bosses and the need for IVF in the upcoming months. Dr. McBride had sent all our records over to Hartland Medical, and our first appointment was in two weeks. The information that was provided to us in anticipation of that visit was intense. It looked like frequent visits, constant monitoring, and the ability to change expectations and treatment on a dime. Flexibility wasn't my strong suit; Case in point: how I reacted to Bill and Mike closing up shop a little over a year ago. Plus, I wasn't sure how my bosses would take me, saying, "Hey! Change of plans, another doctor's appointment tomorrow, even though I just had one today!" Hartland Medical was roughly an hour and a half north of us—almost a straight shot up I-91. That was a minimum of three hours in the car each visit, provided that we didn't hit morning or evening commute traffic. Then there was the actual visit time. I had no idea what I was getting into, and I felt like I didn't know how to prepare myself, or my bosses, for this upcoming commitment.

As I pulled up our office messenger, I saw the red circle next to my boss's name disappear and change back into a green dot, indicating he was off the phone. I took some calming breaths and rushed across the office to grab him before he was sucked into another meeting. When I arrived at his office, my manager was closing the door to chat privately with him. My shoulders slumped. Partially in relief, procrastinating is the name of the game after all, but also in an overwhelming sense of dread. Waiting wasn't a strength of mine, either.

I turned around and headed to a coworker's office for some chitchat while keeping my eye on his office door. After five minutes, I saw Jameson, the manager, open the door and hover, offering a few parting words to Landon. I quickly ended my small talk and hoofed it across the office, hoping to snag both of them.

Clearly, my nerves were showing on my face because Jameson did a double take before asking, "Hey, everything okay?"

"Yeah," I assured him halfheartedly. "Can I borrow you and Landon for a quick minute?"

"Sure."

He followed me back into Landon's office and took the chair by the door. I walked further in and took the one directly across from Landon's desk. I tapped my heel and clasped my hands neatly in front of me. Landon looked at me, eyebrows furrowed, and glanced quickly at Jameson before looking back to me.

I jumped in. "So, uh, Josh and I have been trying to have a baby for two years now." Landon blinked but otherwise showed no reaction. "And obviously, it hasn't happened." I gestured lamely at my very-not-pregnant stomach. "So we've been doing all sorts of tests and consults, and we were told last month that if we ever want kids, we'll have to get them through IVF." I inhaled deeply and said the next part quickly. "If IVF even works. It has like a 30-40% success rate, so even then, it's not a guarantee."

Jameson leaned forward. "Jesus, sorry about that. That's rough." His voice was quiet and super nice. He and his wife had agreed years ago that they never wanted children, which was cool with them, but he said it in such a way that even though he couldn't empathize with what I was going through, he could sympathize. I looked over at him, nodded silently in thanks, swallowed, and turned back to Landon.

"So, I'm telling you this because we start the IVF process next week. Our first visit is already on the calendar, but all future visits are completely subject to change. I might have to go in every day, every other day, every three days. It's a complete unknown. And the clinic is up north in Lebanon. So it's an hour and a half there and the same coming back." I trailed off.

"So, I'm guessing you'll be missing work for these appointments?" Landon asked. His mustache slightly wiggled as he spoke.

I forced my heel to stop bouncing and to project calm. "Yes, I'll be missing work. And I'm not sure the dates or times of the appointments either. So I just wanted to let you know."

Landon looked at me blankly, like he couldn't understand why I was telling him this.

I waited.

He broke it. "Well, obviously, you need to do what you need to do for your family. We 100% support you. Let us know what you need from us during this time, and we'll do our best to make it happen. Having kids was the greatest thing that ever happened to me, and luckily we didn't have to go down that route, but I hear about many people that do. Who knows, maybe it will happen by accident later. You hear stories all the time of people who do IVF and get pregnant naturally later."

I cringed slightly at the commonly uttered reassurance. I shared our IVF journey with my softball teammates this past week, and Josh had updated his family and his work. Naturally, everyone was super supportive, but they all uttered similar sentiments to my boss. I'm sure people used these sayings because they thought it made the infertile person feel better. But it didn't. Anytime I heard or read things like that, those empty assurances, the ones that made it seem like infertility was just a minor inconvenience that could be fixed by time or by 'not trying,' I wanted to scream. If literal medical professionals told us it would not happen without IVF, what makes Joe Schmoe off the streets with an English degree so sure that we would get pregnant by not trying? Like, the act of not thinking about it magically fixes my husband's cysts and gives him oodles of sperm to spare? Not likely. They meant well, but hearing stories about someone's friend from high school doing IVF and getting triplets and then another friend doing IVF twelve times before giving up, while anecdotally interesting, were **not** stories I wanted to hear when entering this unknown phase of our pursuit of parenthood.

"Yeah, Ashley, of course, we support you guys. Let us know if you need anything, and we'll be behind you 100%." Jameson echoed Landon's words.

The conversation was going much better than I had dreamed. I felt my shoulder tension lessen as I realized they would not give me a hard time. I was mustering up a response to Jameson when Landon interrupted with a question that threw me off a little.

"What is IVF anyway? Is that when they stick the thing up you and inject some donor stuff into you?" That vague and slightly yucky interpretation of fertility treatments gave me pause. I figured he knew what IVF was. It didn't occur to me that I might tell people we were doing IVF, and they might not know what it was. I'd lived in the fertility world for so long that I forgot that not everyone lived and breathed the acronyms and vocabulary.

"No, Landon. Jesus." Jameson choked out. As an atheist, he said "Jesus" a lot. The irony there was funny enough to bring me back to the task.

"Sort of. They'll basically be injecting me with lots of drugs that force me to ovulate. The drugs will act as turbo shots to my ovaries and reproductive system, so rather than only producing one or two follicles or eggs to be fertilized, like a normal woman would in any month, the drugs are supposed to make it, so I produce more than that. They'll monitor me to make sure I'm responding well to the drug cocktail, and then they'll go in and suck the eggs out of me with a large, scary needle. Then they'll then take a sperm sample from Josh and under a microscope, choose the sperm that looks the best, and use a super small needle to shoot those little suckers into the eggs they retrieved. One sperm to one egg. Then, over the course of four to six days, they'll monitor the eggs to see which ones remain viable and turn into embryos. Apparently, the attrition rate is a little depressing." I gave a lopsided half smile, my left side of my mouth turning up slightly. "Then, from there, they can take the healthy embryos that survived those few days and inject them back into my uterus. Next you just hope that they are "sticky embryos" and stick to my uterus. Two weeks later, you go back for bloodwork and hope you're sprinkled in baby dust and get some joyful news!"

"Two weeks? You must wait for two entire weeks before finding out whether it works?"

"From what I've read on the community boards, it's called The Two Week Wait (TWW), and apparently it's absolute torture."

"Well, yeah. After waiting for as long as you have, waiting two more weeks probably doesn't seem like much when you're sitting here discussing it, but I'm sure it's brutal when you're living it."

"Yeah, there are online lists of things you can do during the wait to make it not seem painfully slow."

Landon chimed in, "and you can't take a home test during that time?"

"No, you can. It's just not as reliable. The hospital advises everyone to wait. For several reasons. But there are lots of people that don't and test at home."

"Yes, I can see you doing that." Jameson smiled at me–knowing me so well already, even though I hadn't even worked there for a full year.

"The amount of money that I've spent on pregnancy tests would make you sick," I confirmed. "I finally did a Subscribe and Save on Amazon. They aren't super great tests like First Response or anything name brand like that. But they're good enough."

"So, how is what you said different from what I said?" Landon queried.

I paused, looked at Jameson, and then back to Landon. He was almost seventy years old and had a very dry sense of humor. I wasn't quite sure if he was messing with me or asking. I forced out a little chuckle and smiled at him, patting my thighs with finality. "Okay then. I just wanted to give you guys a heads up that that's what's been going on with me, and that's what's going to be going on with me." My tongue tripped over my messy sentence, but I got it out.

"Not a problem. Again, we support you. Do what you need to do for your family. Family always comes first."

"I appreciate that, Landon."

"Of course."

As I stood up to leave, I waited by the door for Jameson to walk out with me, but he remained seated.

"Go ahead. I have to stay and chat with Landon. Can you shut the door behind you?" Figuring they were going to discuss what I had just told them, I nodded silently, gave them a smile of thanks, and shut the door softly behind me. The relief I felt from their calm acceptance and support was nearly overwhelming. I partly wanted to cry from relief, partly wanted to take back every nasty thought I had during tax season for working extra and receiving not even a thank you, and partly wanted to call Hartland Medical and ask for an earlier appointment. Instead, I just rushed back to my desk to tell Josh he was right; they were totally supportive like he said they'd be.

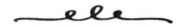

Josh and I celebrated the start of our IVF week with a round of golf before a low-key dinner at the local brewery. To say we were excited was an understatement. No more tests, just action. Going forward. Moving onward towards our baby goal. And that eagerly awaited appointment was this upcoming week. Another tax season was over, and we were looking at starting our summer with some IVF and a side of relaxation.

I ordered my signature grilled cheese without tomato, french fries, and chocolate milk. The waitress looked at me like I was nuts, but I was used to that; my diet of a five-year-old had never steered me wrong before. There was never a risk that I wouldn't like what I ordered. My nickname was Risk-Averse Ashley. Not really, but it could have been.

The waitress walked away from the table toward the bar area, where they had a collection of TVs suspended from the ceiling, all airing different channels. The subtitles flew across the screen in stark relief against the visual backdrops. I looked back to Josh as he picked up where he left off when she came to take our order. "Then Chris tells me they need him to do a semen analysis but never told him that there isn't a room at the clinic for him to do it in."

"Same as they did to you!"

"Yes! The difference is that Chris lives even further away and can't go home, do it, and come back in to drop it off. Too long of a car ride for the sample."

"Did you tell him he could use our house?"

"Of course. He declined, though. Said it was too weird. Then he tells me he just did it in his truck in the parking lot!"

"No!" I gasped out.

Josh laughed hysterically. "Yes! The guy just got into his truck and just rubbed one out right there in the back lot!"

"Oh my God!" I joined in, tears leaking from my eyes. "No!"

He banged on the table with his hand and leans forward, resting his forehead on his arm, his shoulders heaving. I pick up my water to take a sip, think better of it given the laughs still wracking my body, and place it back down, sip not taken. Our friends Chris and Jamie had not had any luck in the procreating game since we last saw them. They were approaching five or six months, and I don't know how she did it, but Jamie was able to get her doctor to see her earlier than the one-year mark. She wasn't thirty yet, so I wasn't sure how she managed it, but she was direct enough with the doctors, and she wasn't making the same mistakes I did. Whatever she did, she got shit done. Case in point, Chris getting a semen analysis done before more invasive testing on her.

"Oh my God," I laughed again as another wave of giggles hit me. "Can you imagine if he was caught?"

"I guess he could just try to blame the hospital for not giving him a room?"

"That's got to be a felony. Or illegal. Or something!"

"One would think," Josh agreed.

I wiped my eyes again with the palms of my hands and looked back toward the bar area. I blinked. My head jerked back, and I blinked harder to clear my vision.

"What the heck?" I murmur. "What the heck?" I say louder. "Josh! Do you see the news?" My stomach clenched, and I couldn't believe my eyes.

"What?" He whipped his head around to the tv area and looked around.

"Did you see this?" I semi-shouted, gesturing wildly at the tv screen towards the end of the bar.

"No." He took a sharp breath.

Staring at us from the TV screen was a news story from a local channel announcing that Hartland Medical's IVF program was being closed, effective immediately.

"This can't be real," I whispered, fully in shock.

"Did they give a reason?" Josh leaned closer and squinted at the tiny captions. "Blah, blah, blah... lack of staffing. Are you shitting me!" He exclaimed.

"This can't be happening." I was still not functioning completely.

"Did they call you? Did they tell you they were going to be canceling their IVF center?" I shook my head. "Why in the world would they not call us?" He swore swiftly and with a lot of color.

"Obviously, they didn't call me!" I bit out. "I would have told you!" I took in a shuddering breath. "I can't believe they didn't tell us. We were supposed to start this week. *This week*!" I ended with a cry. Then the dam broke, and the tears came pouring down. Josh came around the table, threw his arms around me, and rocked me back and forth softly. I couldn't believe our luck. Sometimes it was hard not to look into this and feel like this was the universe's way of telling us this wasn't meant to be.

I took a few shaky breaths and tried to get myself under control. We were getting looks from the patrons next to us, but I couldn't find it in me to care all that much. I clung to Josh and slowly regulated my breathing while searching the table for a napkin to blow my nose. When I was done, Josh let me go and went back around the table to sit down.

"Okay, first things first. We need to call the clinic and ask what the fuck is going on. We also need to research other IVF clinics in our area. Or maybe that should be first. The hospital probably won't answer us after hours. Yeah, so first, we research. Then we call. Finally, we call McBride and have them do a new referral. "

"Josh," I started dejectedly, "I've already researched IVF clinics near us. The next closest is in Springfield, Massachusetts. It's about the same distance away. It's just out of state, so I don't know how insurance treats that."

"Well, we can look into that. This isn't the end of the world." Unflappable, Josh rallies again.

"What are all of their IVF patients doing right now? What if they were mid-cycle?" I couldn't help but wonder.

"I'm sure they were referred somewhere or taken care of somehow. Maybe they're just closed for future patients and will see the current patients through the end of their active cycles?"

"I would hope so!"

"Jeez. What a clusterfuck."

We received a sharp look from an older lady at a table next to us. I shot her a small smile in apology, even though I'm sure it rang false, and looked back to Josh.

"Okay, so we'll look at other clinics and get the lay of the land on what our next steps are. I'll see what McBride suggests and I'll call insurance tomorrow too." I waited for Josh's nod and finished with, "no big deal, we can handle this."

Maybe if I repeated it enough times to myself, I'd finally believe it.

Fifteen

It was May 24, and we were heading to our two-hour IVF orientation at Burr Medical in Springfield, Massachusetts. After Hartland closed their IVF clinic, Dr. McBride moved quickly to get all our records sent to the next closest facility that had what we were looking for. Like every step so far, the closing of Hartland seemed like the end of the world at the time but ended up delaying us only about a week. I made a mental note to remember that and to take that lesson to heart. When you're in it, living it, everything seems so fresh and overwhelming, but once you step back, it seems much more inconsequential. I was going to adopt a broader worldview going forward; I had a feeling that I'd need some perspective to get through the next few months.

After driving the hour and a half down into Massachusetts, we were amazed when our map app took us to a place that looked more like a castle from Northern Ireland than a hospital. It had towers. Literal towers. We made an obvious Hogwarts joke while admiring the view. Made entirely of brick and stone, with windows peppering the side facing us, it looked like it had seen some winters. Just counting the windows from the ground, we counted nine different floors. Which, coming from our small-town hospital, was seriously impressive. As we parked the car and walked toward the specified entrance per the email instructions, the building loomed over us. The surrounding hardscape is a stark contrast to home but also a little intimidating. This was a place that saw thousands and thousands of people on a very regular basis. Who were we? On the one hand, they had a robust infertility program. But I also didn't want to just become a number to them.

I shook off the sense of foreboding and pulled up the instructions again, navigating us to the classroom that would host our orientation class

They handed us a three-ring binder that was stuffed with IVF background. At two inches thick, the supporting documents inside tested the limits of the metal rings. We found a seat towards the middle and flicked through the pages while we waited for everything to start.

We blew through the first few pages. Mission statements, the itinerary for today's IVF Overview Class, parking instructions, directions to the other buildings, and the financial services contact information didn't interest us (at the current moment). Instead, I flipped until we saw an IVF Checklist. At the top, in bold, it outlined all the prerequisites that we must complete before beginning the IVF process. We looked through the list, taking turns making notes on what we knew was already done and what things we weren't sure about. When finished with that page, I flipped until we arrived at the table of contents.

"Dear Lord. No wonder this class is two hours long," I muttered to Josh. It was three full pages of subjects that would be discussed tonight. A lot I already knew from research, but as Josh only ever really listened to my findings under duress, and I imagine others here were like him, I could see why there would need to be a well-planned lesson plan for this visit. I was tempted to ask if I could just take the test already and test out of sitting through it. When I saw the stern-looking doctor enter the room and head over to the IVF coordinator, I thought better of my joke. Probably not the right place or time.

The IVF coordinator stepped forward once the first couple found their seats and settled in. "Good afternoon. I'm in charge of managing the IVF clinic here at Burr Medical. We welcome you all here today and look forward to working with you, even if it is under circumstances that might not be ideal. Our job is to help coordinate your cycle and implement your physician's plan for you. We'll discuss the various available protocols and all aspects of your cycle, including timing, scheduling, medication mixing and administration, and how you will be monitored. There will be a ton of information tonight, some of which you are bound to forget, but we're always just a phone call or email away."

I pulled a pen out of my purse and eagerly awaited her next words. I was a total nerd, always had been. Taking notes, listening to an authority figure teach something? Right up my alley, I looked over at Josh in excitement—we were finally here! He glanced down at my pen, took in my eager expression, and rolled his eyes with a slight hitch on the left side of his mouth. I looked forward again.

"As a reminder, you need to complete all the diagnostic tests included at the beginning of this package before you can begin treatment with us. Also, we require a pre-authorization from your insurance company. For those that are out of state, if you need support from us, we'll be happy to assist you. But please be aware that the referral needs to come from your PCP, not a related fertility specialist that may have sent you here."

I wrote the words "Pre-authorization?" in messy letters at the top of my page.

"We do ultrasounds daily at our main office on a first-come, first serve basis. Come upstairs, add your name to the clipboard at the desk when you arrive, and we'll work our way down the line. Please indicate whether you are here to receive an ultrasound and/or bloodwork on the clipboard. We do our best to work through everyone as quickly and as thoroughly as possible. Please try stressing to your employers that there are no guarantees on the timing of anything during this process. The lab opens up one hour earlier than we do, at seven, so if you would like to check in with us and then go downstairs for bloodwork while you wait, that is a common practice—do whatever you think is best. We need the bloodwork done no later than nine, so we can have your results back in time for our daily protocol review. This allows us to determine if changes are needed to your medications."

I swallowed. No scheduled appointments? That seemed like a recipe for anarchy.

"In Vitro fertilization involves stimulating the ovaries, removing multiple eggs, fertilizing the eggs in the lab, culturing the embryos in the incubators, and then transferring the embryos into the uterus. Assisted reproductive technology has undergone vast developments in the last several years. Here at Burr Medical, we see success rates that are right on par, even slightly higher than average. In section one, you'll see our success rates for each age group and per cycle type. Cycle success rates when using fresh embryos range from eleven to thirty-five percent. You can see the swing primarily depends on the age of the woman. Cycle success rates when using frozen embryos are higher—in the thirty to forty-five percent range. Last year alone, we completed roughly 300 fresh cycles and almost 200 frozen cycles. We try to steer patients away from multiple embryo transfers, so you'll see that our live singleton occurrences outweigh our twin occurrences. The risks increase when you transfer more than one embryo, but your assigned physician will discuss with you during your specific protocol meetings and will work with you to determine the proper course of action."

She flipped through some slides on the screen, and then the success rates were displayed starkly. I breathed a sigh of relief once again that we figured this out now rather than waiting until after thirty or thirty-five years old. The drop-off in success rates was staggering. She spoke some more about risk factors and unique traits that could affect outcomes. As she referred us to sources for smoking cessation, weight loss support, and other services, I let my mind wander and skimmed ahead a few pages. They brought me back to reality when I heard, "Does anyone have questions so far?"

The insurance coordinator continued on about the process and expectations, the holidays and protocols, insurance, and counseling. I scribbled furiously on my margins when I had questions and starred the ones that needed to be asked immediately.

"We individualize each cycle according to your response. Sometimes it will require you to come to us daily, though that is rare. However, you must be prepared for that if it's required. After taking the stimulation drugs, in the next three to five days, you'll be required to come in to start monitoring your follicular development by ultrasound. You'll also start your bloodwork then. Frequently monitoring your blood levels is our way of checking your estradiol and progesterone levels to ensure we don't need to tweak your doses. It also provides an estimation of ovarian response and follicular maturation. Once your follicles appear nearly mature based on that bloodwork and the ultrasounds, you will be told to administer your hCG Trigger Shot to induce final follicular maturation." She paused and looked at us severely. "Now listen carefully. Most of your medications have a window of administration. You can administer them within a one to two-hour swing most days, so make sure you pick a time that can be repeated for quite a while. But the Trigger Shot needs to be timed exactly. I repeat," she looked around almost angrily, "exactly, thirty-six hours before your egg retrieval. Early or later triggering may adversely affect your egg quality or numbers."

I wrote my notes quickly and underlined them several times, emphasizing the word "exactly" on my page.

"The day of your egg retrieval will probably be a day of recovery. You'll be completely under, and they will guide a needle into your vagina. It will then puncture the follicle walls and collect the eggs. Plan on going home and resting. You may be sleepy from the anesthesia and may experience bleeding and cramping. Of course, as you would expect, there are risks from IVF. The egg retrieval process provides the highest risk as there could be bleeding, infection, scar tissue formation, and injury to organs. These risks are rare, but it is still a possibility. Please discuss all concerns with your physician. We would like to address Ovarian Hyperstimulation or OHSS during this class. It's not uncommon when using gonadotropins for IVF. It consists of mild abdominal discomfort five to seven days after hCG administration. However, these symptoms can become severe. In severe cases, there will be massive enlargement and swelling of the ovaries, causing the ovaries to twist, which could result in the need for additional surgery to manage it. You also may develop fluid in your abdominal cavity or chest, making it hard to breathe, and in extremely rare cases, you could develop thromboembolism. If the fluid buildup is intense, we can drain it, but we do our best to monitor your cycles so this doesn't occur."

She blew through some more slides on the screen, generally scaring the pants off me the more she spoke. She discussed the fertilization process more and timelines, cycle cancellations, and various types of miscarriages and then brought it back to negative Nancy land by saying, "and of course, let's discuss ovarian cancer."

I looked at Josh sharply. He frowned quickly before looking forward again.

"The risk of ovarian cancer seems partly related to the number of times a woman ovulates. Therefore, birth control pill use generally decreases that risk. Conversely, infertility treatments increase the risk. Controversial data exists that the ovulation associated with the stimulation drugs may contribute to the risk of future ovarian cancer. There is still a lot of ongoing research about this, especially when pregnancy and breastfeeding tend to decrease ovarian cancer risks. But it is something that you'll need to consider if you have a family history of ovarian cancer."

She paused for questions, but at this point, we were all fairly speechless and properly cowed by this downer of a talk.

"So let's talk transfer day!" She clapped her hands together sharply and did a Jekyll and Hyde mood swing. "Depending on whether you're doing a fresh or frozen transfer, your build-up to transfer day will change, but it is an exciting and wonderful day. Hopefully, the day that you all will become parents! It is a brief procedure that takes place in the OR. We pry open your cervix, guide the catheter upwards, and inject the embryo. There might be slight discomfort as your cervix is opened, but it should be nothing like the egg retrieval surgery. We will prescribe you Valium to help you tolerate the procedure if necessary. Nine days later, you'll come back for a blood test, a beta hCG, and you'll continue with your estrogen and progesterone until we say otherwise—no matter what. I can't stress that enough. If you stop your hormones, you will have a pregnancy loss. The estrogen and the progesterone are the only things supporting the pregnancy in a frozen cycle, so you will miscarry if you stop those drugs."

I scribbled and underlined furiously on my sheet of paper.

She discussed genetic tests and screenings, follow-up appointments, embryo freezing, nonviable pregnancies, and fetal reductions. She emphasized that bleeding was common during IVF cycles and usually came from the cervix or vagina as the progesterone irritates the tissues. She stressed we shouldn't be concerned that it was affecting what was happening inside our uterus, but if it became heavy, similar to a period, we were to call them asap."

She continued on through the rest of the slides as Josh, and I sat there in awe. I obviously had researched IVF to death before coming, but even so, this information was overwhelming. To Josh, who had no baseline, it was even worse. I took out a new sheet and compiled my notes and questions on it, so I wouldn't need to flip through the two hundred other pages to find my questions. As I reviewed my questions, I realized a lot was specific to me and that they might not apply to everyone else. No one else around me needed to hear me ask about asthma risks during IVF or if we could do the bloodwork back home and fax our results to Burr. No one needed to know if I needed to continue my bromocriptine or how to manage my cycles, as I had irregular periods and couldn't plan for them. Instead, I made notes of which I should ask privately with my assigned physician and just marked the ones that were generic enough to be answered here. As she paused for questions at the end, I shot my hand up and started at the beginning, "in parentheses, it says that the partner needs to do a semen analysis here at Burr. We've done a ton of those. Does he need to do another here, or can you just take the results from any of the other tests?" I saw several nods around the room as others agreed with my question.

"I'm sorry, no, the semen analysis needs to be done here with our own specialized and trained lab technicians."

"Okay," I replied and wrote her response in my notes. I muttered "good grief" to Josh as she moved on to someone else.

Sure enough, we stayed the entire two hours, and I felt like we could have stayed even longer. We met the three doctors that oversaw the IVF program at Burr and were told that we'd be assigned to one of them throughout our IVF journey. Nevertheless, depending on the day, they might not be the ones doing our retrievals or transfers just because they managed our cycle and protocols.

My head was spinning as Josh, and I packed up and walked to the car. That was a lot of information to digest. Josh was silent as well. Silence surrounded us as we started the car and pulled out onto I91. Finally, I said, "wow."

"Yeah." He agreed. "If you don't feel comfortable doing this, just say so. It's not my body that has to go through all that. It's yours. If you feel unsafe doing it, I won't pressure you. I just want you to be safe and happy."

"I know," I assured him. "I know. The reward outweighs the risk. I'm 100% confident of that."

"If you say so. If it ever changes, let me know."

Gosh. I loved my guy.

"I know, dear." I reached over and patted his hand with mine. "I know. Love you."

His fingers wrapped tight around my own as he glared out the windshield, "love you too."

Sixteen

I SPENT MOST OF the next day completely distracted at work. I brought my three-ring binder into my office and went line by line down the prerequisites. We had an appointment the following morning with the physician assigned to our case, and I wanted to leave no stone unturned. I wanted to make sure all of my ducks were in a row before arriving so we could get everything started as soon as possible.

So far, the biggest issue was the cross-border referral.

Because I had never met my PCP, things became a little tricky. I was a relatively healthy person, not counting my asthma and infertility, and with the turnover at the clinic, my PCP was changed almost yearly. So whenever I had a checkup, I saw whatever practitioner was available. For instance, when I first met with my OBGYN to start the 'we're trying to conceive' conversation, it was at the same hospital as my PCP, so it didn't seem like an issue that I didn't see my PCP first. She referred me to other doctors and procedures that were done within the same hospital. Again, easy peasy. Then, the OBGYN referred me to Dr. McBride in Vermont. My insurance allowed that and didn't give me any issues. But once again, not once during this process did I call my PCP.

So when I tried calling my PCP's office at the clinic, they were perplexed. The receptionist kept asking if I wanted to make an appointment to see my PCP or if I needed a referral to an OBGYN or a referral to a fertility specialist. After fifteen minutes of being interrupted, put on hold, and then interrupted again, I finally convey enough of my situation that they realized I was already where I needed to be. I just needed a formal referral from the PCP herself rather than a referral from someone who was referred by someone who was referred by someone else.

Long story short–I was directed to a completely different office because, apparently, referrals aren't done by the PCP.

Instead, I had to call the referral line, do the same song and dance all over again, and then submit the request for a referral. They said they'd prepare it and send it to the PCP for review. At this point, I was sweating because my first appointment was the very next day...*tomorrow*. I was promised that it could be backdated if necessary. So I was trying my darndest not to stress.

But, I am me, so stress I did.

I also spent a significant chunk of my day poring over my Explanation of Health Insurance Benefits. I scoured every page of that document and found my insurance, by an act of God, actually covered fertility diagnoses, which we knew, and it also would cover up to six cycles of IVF! I couldn't believe our luck. Just last year, I was devastated about being let go when the firm was being sold, but if I hadn't been given the boot, I would never have found this new job with the very rare IVF benefit.

Thank God.

While requesting the referral, I had the IVF binder in front of me and ran the numbers on my calculator. Under the Financial Considerations section, I compared the numbers to see what we would have to face if we didn't have insurance for IVF. IVF itself was $6,850. IVF with ICSI, where they don't let the sperm invade the mother-ship egg but, instead, insert the chosen guy directly into the egg with a needle, was $8,220. If over ten were injected, the price was raised to $9,109. Each Frozen Embryo Cycle was $2,300. And, if paying out of pocket, payment would need to be received before the start of the cycle. In bold, they stated, '**Visa and MasterCard are accepted.**'

Gee, thanks.

Additional charges included assisted hatching (which would be done before transferring), semen freeze costs, storage of frozen semen, and storage of frozen embryos.

Also in bold was "This does not include the cost of medications."

Holy moly. I knew IVF was expensive, but this was rough. How in the world were two people who weren't an engineer and an accountant supposed to afford this? Because they wouldn't have $15,000 to spend on various infertility tests and subsequent treatment, did that make them less qualified to have a child of their own? Obviously not. But this price was steep. As it was, if we had to pay for this out of pocket... well, we just wouldn't be able to at this point. We drained a sizeable chunk of our savings just to get here. And student loan payments for Josh, house bills, and vehicle payments weren't cheap.

I shot another 'thank you' out into the universe for the health insurance coverage that was allowing this to even be a thing for us.

An exceptional thing about public accounting is that the summers can be flexible. So even though I spent a fair amount of my day trying to get everything sorted, I could work late that night to make up for that time. By the time I left work on Thursday night, I was sitting at thirty-seven hours for the week, and with tomorrow being Friday and having the doctor's appointment down in Massachusetts, I was choosing to head home and mentally prepare.

I had the hardest time falling asleep that night–I just couldn't get comfortable. To make things worse, Josh was sleeping like an absolute baby next to me. Snoring away. Completely oblivious to my unrest.

I wasn't entirely sure why I was so anxious. I knew we were doing this. I knew things were progressing. But a small part of me was worked up–for no discernable reason. When I finally fell asleep, constant waking plagued me and had me frantically checking my phone-worried that I overslept or that my alarm never went off. Saying that I was drowsy on the monotonous drive down to Springfield would be a safe assumption.

The monitoring visits were at a different facility than the orientation visit. A small off-ramp from the highway led us into a somewhat deserted-looking part of town. We parked in the parking garage and strolled towards the entrance. Hardly anyone was here this early in the morning. We made our way through the lobby and up to the third floor. I went to sign in on the clipboard and there were already two names on the list in front of us. I made a mental note to make sure that we left a little earlier next time.

We sat in the small waiting area and looked around curiously. The walls were vibrant orange, the carpet a worn-down blue. Dark mahogany furniture filled up the room somewhat haphazardly. I flipped through several magazines stored on the side table while we waited. Josh just tilted his head back in signature fashion and took a snooze.

After about twenty minutes, we were called back and escorted into a meeting room—no exam room for us this visit. The nurse and medical student went over our medical histories. They confirmed the various tests we had done to date, which we needed to redo here at Burr Medical, and several other housekeeping items.

We were then walked across the hall to the physician's office to go over everything again. Except this time, she outlined what she believed to be the best IVF protocol for our situation.

I was assigned the creatively named 'Birth Control Pill-Lupron Protocol.'

"Because of your irregular menstrual cycles, we give you the birth control pill to help regulate your cycle so we can control the Lupron start date. You'll be on the pill for one month, and then on the first day of your cycle, please call our IVF nurse clinic line. They'll be able to instruct you on the next steps and the important dates of that cycle."

"So, you guys don't know if a particular couple will start a cycle on any given month?" I was incredulous.

"That's correct."

My head jerked, and I blinked dumbly at her. The physician assigned to our case was about fifty years old and had pin-straight brown hair. She whispered and gave the impression of a very calming bedside manner. From the reviews online, people seemed to really love her. But then again, each of the doctors at this clinic received glowing praise, so we really couldn't go wrong.

"How do you plan for a person's cycle?" I was still stuck on the fact that any given month, they could have twenty different couples decide to do IVF, and they would have no way to adjust or plan for that.

"IVF isn't as common as it feels right now. We see roughly 500 IVF patients per year, and a half of those are just frozen cycle patients–where we're just monitoring them and then defrosting their chosen embryo or embryos and transferring. Frozen cycles are much less intense than the fresh transfers with retrievals."

I nodded along even though I was still skeptical that a system like this was sustainable. But what did I know? They'd been doing this for years. I was a total noob. Clearly, it was working for them, despite the fact that there were no scheduled appointments or scheduled cycles.

"We'll have to do an ICSI IVF cycle for you two. Our orientation should have explained this, but rather than taking the sperm sample and depositing it in a culture with the retrieved egg, we select each sperm based on morphology and health and use a very tiny needle to inject that specific sperm into your egg. When the male sperm sample isn't as robust as it should be, ICSI, or Intracytoplasmic Sperm Injection, is the best practice. After this insemination, the cycle is monitored, like a normal IVF cycle. I have the paperwork here that you need to sign and bring back for your next visit." She handed up some forms. "This outlines that ICSI is used to increase the chance of fertilization, but the success rates with ICSI are slightly lower than for conventional insemination. There also are reported statistics that suggest that there is an increased risk of genetic defects in offspring reported. There's a bunch of other information in there for you to review, but once you've looked, we require your signed consent to the procedure." She paused and looked at us, giving us a chance to chime in. When we were silent, she continued, "That is the only difference in the ICSI process. We then put the inseminated egg under a strict monitoring protocol where we check for fertilization. If they fertilize, because not all of them do, we culture them and let them grow for two to six days. Once they've reached the blastocyst stage, we then do the transfer or freeze them for a future cycle."

"What would require us not to do a fresh cycle?" Josh asked.

"Some patients just don't want to or aren't ready. Some have extras they want to use at a later date or possibly donate, either to someone else or to science. Others develop hyperstimulation or are just exhausted from their retrieval and need a break. Some want to do a service called PGS or PGD, which is testing on the remaining embryos, to test for things like chromosomal abnormalities. This information can be very important for certain groups of IVF candidates, as they may be more prone to embryos with abnormalities. Rather than transferring embryos that we know aren't sustainable, we can choose more suitable embryos to transfer." She paused briefly again as if she was debating with herself internally. "A consequence of doing PGS testing is that the report also includes information on whether the embryo is a female or male embryo. We don't make gender selections here at Burr Medical unless it is very specific circumstances, but mostly, we don't let patients pick which embryos we transfer."

Could they do that? That piqued my interest.

"Is the testing covered by insurance as well?"

She gave me a cautious look. Like she was trying not to show a reaction.

"It depends on your insurance and diagnosis, but unless it's medically necessary, usually no."

"And, for us, It's not medically necessary?" I asked leadingly.

"Correct. You don't have any markers that would lend us to believe it is necessary. You're under thirty-seven, neither of you has a history of genetic diseases, and you have no history of recurrent miscarriages or failed IVF cycles." She didn't seem to want me to think about this further.

But I was a dog with a bone.

"How much does it cost out of pocket?"

No harm in asking...

"Last I checked, the lab that we work with charges $1,950 for the testing." She looked at Josh and then back at me. "But again, we're not recommending that for you, as we have no reason to believe that you'd benefit from this testing."

My mind was racing though. The thought of doing a cycle and transferring a dud embryo, then having to do everything all over again–and enduring another round of the waiting game–was abhorrent to me. I didn't want to risk that and a small part of me was super interested in knowing what the sex of the baby was before they even transferred it. I knew some people wanted their babies' sex to be a surprise, but at this point, just *having* a baby would be a surprise.

I was over surprises.

"Noted." Josh chimed in - ever the peacekeeper. He already knew where my mind was heading.

She rallied herself from knowing that I was down a mental rabbit hole and soldiered on, handing us more forms and instructions. On one sheet was a silhouette of a woman with random areas filled in with gray hash lines. "These are the acceptable injection sites. You'll find many tips and tricks on the web about administering the shots. Please don't do them. Instead, follow the instructions in our pamphlets or the videos we've provided. However, you can use those tips and tricks to deal with the itching, burning, etc., you may feel after administering the shot."

Heck, some discomfort while taking a shot and after it? Probably nothing compared to childbirth. Small price to pay for a baby. Easy peasy.

She handed us several more forms while Josh and I sat there, mouths agape. Honestly, I was still wildly unprepared for this process even with all my preparation. The internet only takes you so far. Now that I was here and living it, I was becoming acutely aware of the gaps in my knowledge and experiencing the adage of "you don't know what you don't know."

As she was instructing us on where to go for our blood work and Josh's 100th semen analysis, I scribbled furiously on the margins of my handouts. I also circled the items that I'd have to look into more and then do a follow-up with her after completing my research.

We thanked her for our time and left the office. While passing through the reception area, we saw six other couples waiting, either reading old magazines or playing on their phones.

The lab was on the first floor, and there was standing room only. After standing in line for fifteen minutes to check in, the receptionist asked for my license and told us to take a seat. Luckily, this room had TVs, but the one where we sat was broadcasting in Spanish. We both were pretty good at Spanish in high school and college... but like any muscle, if you don't use it, you lose it. And they were speaking much too fast for me to truly understand.

I noticed that almost everyone around me was speaking in Spanish. I wasn't fully aware, until then, that the demographic in the Springfield area had a large Hispanic presence.

"Hey, maybe by the time this is done, we'll be back to our old Spanish-speaking ways!"

I just rolled my eyes at my ever-the-optimist husband.

After thirty long minutes of eavesdropping and asking each other if we remembered specific words, they finally called my name. I jumped up eagerly, ready to be done and head home when she handed me back my license and a sheet of paper instead.

She pointed to a door behind me that led down another hallway and instructed me to follow it to the chairs at the end.

When I did as she advised, I found it was just the hospital's clever way of splitting up the waiting room. Because now I was still in a waiting room, but it was smaller than the other. So physiologically easier to stomach because I felt like I was closer to being seen. As I sat down, I reviewed the papers received from the IVF Team. In my thoughts, there was a war going on. Did we want to find the money to pay for PGS testing? Would it affect our decision to transfer an embryo at all? Was it even likely that something would be wrong? Was I just being overly cautious by wanting the testing? I was still doing circles in my mind when they called my name.

As the phlebotomist did the first of what would come to be innumerable blood draws, we made small talk. She used a needle that was slightly thicker than my abused veins wanted to handle, and I winced. As I explained about IVF, she nodded with understanding and assured me that next time, she'd use a smaller needle.

After leaving, we pulled into the driveway, Josh parked the car, and we sat there silently for a minute. This was it—our first of many appointments. We discussed the pros and cons of everything on the car ride home and felt we had a good plan forward. Our referral was in place. Our appointment went off without a hitch. We received the protocol, and they put in an order for the medications. I made a mental note to check on delivery and unpack the drugs immediately as some of them had to be refrigerated. I spent a good chunk of the car ride researching organization techniques for

IVF materials, and Josh and I had developed a good storage plan for sorting the various wipes, needles, syringes, and vials. Our first order of business, though, was a nap. We were up super early to drive down there, and both of us had slept like garbage the night before. We'd run into the store later so we could buy the storage containers.

But for now, it was Friday; we had a plan.

And it was time to rest.

Seventeen

"You only have thirty-six hours on your timesheet for last week," One of my managers repeated to me again.

Again, I nodded. But this time, I reiterated, "yes, I know. I'm salary, though. I had a doctor's appointment. This would pick up speed in the coming months. I told you guys. You said not to worry."

"Yes, we did, but we didn't understand the true scope of what this would entail. It seems like you're going to be missing a lot of time going forward."

I felt like I was in the twilight zone. "Yes," I repeated. "It's a major medical procedure. It requires appointments frequently, sometimes daily, depending on how things are going." I paused. "We discussed all this already."

I didn't understand what was happening.

It was Monday morning, and I had just gotten to work. The weekend went great. After setting up our game plan and figuring out our next steps, it took a load from my shoulders, and I could finally get a good sleep. It felt like all was right in the world, and we were moving forward. However, when I arrived in the office, the office manager came to me and started asking me about my timesheet from last week. She said that I was required to take PTO for the time missed while at the doctor's or that she'd have to reduce my pay for the time I missed. I was a little speechless and pretty confused.

Bill's office had never asked me to track anything like that, and as it was my first and only job out of college, I didn't know that it was a departure from the norm.

From my way of thinking, I was a salaried employee. I was paid for the work I did, not the hours worked. I believed I was entitled to be paid the same whether I worked forty-six or thirty-six. I shouldn't have to take my vacation time for a doctor's appointment. I shouldn't have to add time to get up to my forty-hour week. If that were the case, then I'd be hourly. I said this to her, she nodded and said she had to talk to my manager.

And now, here we were.

"Yes, you said that it was going to be a time commitment, but we didn't fully process at the time what that would entail. After discussion with the firm owners, we think maybe you would be better served if we switched you to hourly rather than salary."

Umm, excuse me? What!

She saw the look on my face and kept speaking. "That way, we're only paying you for the time that you're working, and you won't be burdened by trying to rush back into the office to hit your forty hours."

Is this legal? I thought to myself.

Aloud I dragged out, "Okay. But I imagine you're going to make it retroactive so I will be entitled to all the overtime I worked during tax season, at least?"

Crickets.

"No, we'll make it active as of last week, the first week that you didn't hit your forty. I'll need to have you sign some forms, and I need to call the Department of Labor on a couple of things to make sure we're doing this correctly, but I think that's best for everyone."

I felt my face heat and heard my heart pounding in my ears. My chest vibrated with thumps, and I clenched my hands under the table. My frequently jittering foot was dead still as I processed what they were saying to me.

It felt like a betrayal. Their words played on a loop in my mind, "we support you. Do what you need to do. Don't worry about work." The hypocrisy was stinging. I didn't know if I wanted to cry or yell. The hours that I put in this tax season. Some weeks to the point of mental breakdowns, and this was how they treated me in my metaphorical hour of need? I didn't receive a bonus or a raise for those extra hours. But I missed three hours on a Friday for a doctor's appointment, and now I was being switched to hourly? Fuck that. If I were a cartoon character, you would see my engagement meter plummet down into red and wink out with a soft beep.

"Yeah, okay. Get me whatever papers you need to. I'll sign them." I stood up, gave a perfunctory nod, and swiftly left the room before I burst into tears.

I hustled down to my office and shut the door softly. I quickly changed my mind and turned around and back out the door. I went straight to the stairs and down into the parking lot. When I was safely in my car, I called Josh and explained everything that happened. He was just as surprised. He didn't have the feeling of betrayal and hurt that I had. He was more concerned about whether it was even legal to do this. He requested that I call and ask the DOL and that he would do the same. Josh said because I was missing time because of a medical condition, to his way of thinking, maybe switching me to hourly for treatment of the medical condition shouldn't be allowed. Regardless, we'd both call and ask.

We disconnected.

As I sat there in my car talking to various DOL agents and texting Josh with updates, I got myself under control. I was hurt and felt betrayed by this, but could understand why a business owner wouldn't want to pay for someone to go to IVF appointments. It would be a drain on resources with no financial return. Especially in public accounting when you're billed by the hour. Recognizing these feelings gave me a sense of freedom. I used to want to time my baby making a round tax season so my employer wouldn't feel the impact of me being on maternity leave during tax season. But honestly, if this was their attitude, then it didn't matter when I had my baby. I should stop feeling guilty for wanting to have a baby and breaking my back to schedule around a time that was 'convenient' for my employer.

Even one that I enjoyed working for.

The DOL agent affirmed they were allowed to switch me to hourly, as long as they didn't switch me back to salary for tax season. It flabbergasted me that this was on the up and up, but by now, I was resigned to my fate. I told myself I would make mad bank next tax season if I worked the same hours as I did this most recent one. So maybe being switched to hourly would be a good thing.

If we continued to struggle and I had to miss even more time... Then I'd really be missing the unlimited sick time I had at Bill's firm.

Don't know what you got till it's gone.

As the day dragged on, I forced myself to come to terms with this new reality until I was back to my usual self. The timing worked out because, as I finally came to grips with my lingering sense of anger, a manager came in with the forms to sign. I pleasantly signed them, not needing to hide the bitterness that was so prevalent that morning and made idle chitchat. The manager happily took the documents, wished me well, and headed out the door. She was completely unaware of how the interaction that morning had entirely broken any loyalty I had to her or the firm and how betrayed I was that someone I admired so much could hurt me so effectively without even realizing it.

Eighteen

"OH MY GOD, JOSH! I feel like Walter White!" I stared at the giant cardboard box in front of me. When I pulled into the driveway earlier and saw the giant box, my heart started racing. As I rushed inside and lugged the box in with me, the excitement of being one step closer to our baby goal was overwhelming.

"Have you opened it?" Josh asked in my ear.

"Yeah, as soon as I got it inside. It's huge - like two by two by two. And filled to the brim with supplies." I paused briefly. "And dry ice." I started pulling out the baggies full of goodies. "There are several bags full of needles and syringes... All different sizes... some vials. Some more vials... and a few more vials. A travel box of some sort. There were boxes for disposing of the needles. Some wipes. Some gauze. More needles. Oh my God!" I shrieked. "These are huge!"

I stared at the needles in horror.

Josh was silent on the other end of the line while I processed the slight fear coursing through my veins.

"Umm, how sure are you that you want a baby?" I asked, half-jokingly. I couldn't tear my eyes away from the offending needles.

Josh coughed quietly in my ear. No doubt getting slightly impatient while I just silently breathed into the phone. I organized the items on the dining room table in front of me. Needles to the right, sorted by size.

Medications in the middle. Refrigerated meds on the top, non-refrigerated closer to me. And gauzes and wipes to the far left.

"Okay," I started again. "I have different-sized needles here. Menopur, Follistim, Lupron, estrogen patches, and progesterone suppositories. I also have papers here that show me different injection sites and the mixing combinations of the drugs."

"Does the paperwork match the videos that they had us watch?" He was referring to a site that the hospital directed us to that outlined the exact mixing and injection steps that we were to follow. There were a few tweaks from the video instructions that they advised us not to follow as the information there was dated, but besides that, the rest was to be taken as gospel.

"Yup. Everything is the same. Actually, the body image printouts are super helpful. It's hash-marked in the areas where you can do the injections. Much better than the vague description of a couple of inches here and a few finger sizes away from there. Wherever here and there are."

"Have you called the clinic yet and asked them about the insurance letter yelling at you?"

I had received a letter from insurance basically chastising me for ordering the drugs from the facility that the fertility clinic recommended. I didn't think it would be an issue that I ordered from the licensed pharmaceutical distributor that literally had the words "fertility pharmacy" in its name. But apparently, that was a big no-no. There was some threatening language that made me worried that the order would be rejected by insurance. So I needed to call up the head nurse asap and figure that out. There were several mortgage payments worth of drugs in front of me. If we were going to need to choke up those funds, then we needed to rearrange our finances a bit. Mostly to the tune of no extra college loan principal payments, no extra car and truck payments, no money into savings that month and no more golfing dates for the rest of the year, just to name a few.

We also experienced a bit of drama a week and a half ago when I was trying to figure out my official period start date. I spotted on June 7, but it was light. Then again, I was constantly spotting. And I didn't know at what point they considered it my official period start date because the rest of my cycle hinged on that Day One. On Day Three, I was to start my birth control pill and go in for baseline bloodwork. But sometimes, my cycle was hard to determine. Sometimes I would spot for a week, then it got heavier, turning into my period. Sometimes it started like a wrecking ball. But do they count the first spotting day as the period starts? Or the first day that is really heavy? How heavy did 'heavy' need to be tampon or pad worthy? Is it pantyliner worthy? Was I overthinking this? Yes. But it caused me heartache the last couple of weeks as I tried to figure this out because so much was riding on this cycle.

So obviously, that had me in knots.

June 27 was here before I knew it, and it was my first night of shots. I was all fired up with nerves. I double and triple-checked the measurements and instructions. Everything was lined up in front of me. Josh and I had discussed our game plan for the shot mixing and injection, and we were good to go.

When it came time for the shot, I found I wasn't so convinced of our plan anymore. We recorded our antics on Josh's phone, so we would have the videos to re-watch later when our child wanted to know how they were conceived and how the process worked. We thought it would be a fun story. Now that I was sitting in front of the camera and pulling up my shirt for Josh to poke me... I felt powerless.

I wasn't in control of anything. And this was yet just another experience that was being done to me. The last few years had been the same. Me being powerless, and I had no agency in my life. I started to panic mildly.

"Uh, no, I'm not ready!" As I swiped his hand away from my belly. "I'm not ready."

I took some deep breaths and girded myself.

"Okay, so change of plans. I'm doing this myself." Maybe if I took control and did it to myself, I'd feel a little less powerless.

"As you wish," he murmured, eyeballing my panicked behavior with a needle in hand warily.

I double-checked the Lupron measurement of ten units. Then, grabbing the alcohol wipe, I obsessively wiped my stomach again. Sigh. I took a couple more calming breaths. My research so far showed that some of these shots tended to hurt. But I could do this. I will do this.

"Okay. In like a dart. Quick jab. Steady plunge. I got this." I psyched myself up. A couple more steadying breaths and...

Ouch. Ouch. Ouch.

Worth every shot, I reminded myself

And it was done.

"You're a badass." Josh smiled at me. "Did it hurt?"

"When I fell from Heaven?" I quipped back.

"Did it?"

"Oh my God. Did we double check we did the correct amount?" My mind started racing with the possibilities.

"Yes, we checked. We have it on video if that would make you feel better. Are you doing okay?"

"Well, I don't feel like I'm hemorrhaging or having a heart attack." I put my finger on my pulse in jest.

"My drama queen." He chuckled fondly. "You did that very, very easily. I'm proud of you."

As he spoke, the area to the right of my belly button got a little itchy. Then it burned.

Yup, it was definitely burning.

"Agh! It's burning!" I patted it and rubbed around the injection site. Josh hopped up and ran to the kitchen to grab an ice pack from the freezer. When I placed it on my belly, I felt instant relief, but the high-anxiety part wondered if I had an allergic reaction. A little hypochondriac moment, but it thankfully passed quickly.

"The good news going forward is that the nurses gave us a one-to-two-hour window to take the shot every night. We'll try to time it for eight o'clock exactly every night, but it's a relief to know that if field hockey or softball or something runs late or we want to catch a movie or something, that it's not the end of the world because of that window. A lot of the information you found said that it had to be exact, so I'm glad it's not like that anymore." Josh rambled to distract me from the itching.

I nodded absently, trying very hard not to rub the injection site, and plopped the needle with its cap into the sharps container.

"Wait, we have a new one of those every single day?" Josh seemed appalled at the waste.

"Yup, and it's going to make for an impressive baby photo when we have all the needles on the ground surrounding our little IVF miracle!" I was already planning the IVF-themed photoshoot. Pinterest was full of great ideas, and I had spent loads of time trying to turn this IVF frown upside down and attempting to make it unique and fun. I had a 'Command Center' created for the IVF supplies on our dining room table. I had a plastic drawer tote thing on the table with syringes in one drawer, gauze and alcohol wipes in another, birth control pills, and other non-refrigerated medications in one drawer. And miscellaneous items in a box to the side. I retyped the calendar given to us by the IVF clinic and wrote the exact doses and the days of each medication. And color-coded each day. I added tentative monitoring visits and other important dates of this cycle, subject to change, and I was ready. The Queen of Organization had struck, and I was as prepared as I'd ever be.

Like I said, I was going to make this as fun!

"That seems sick and twisted to have a baby surrounded by needles." Josh offered his (unwanted) opinion.

"It will be cute. Promise. I'll show you what I have in mind when we're in bed."

"Whatever you want, dear." He acquiesced. Josh often gave me what I wanted. Not because I was spoiled, even though I was, but because he was super easygoing and not much bothered him. So if it didn't bother him, and it was in his power to give it to me, he usually went along with it. I was 100% aware of how lucky I was to have a partner like him.

"Mark the date, Joshy. June 27. The start of our cycle. The start of the, hopefully, last leg of our infertility journey! They say that I'll have cramps, headaches, nausea, and sore boobs from the meds! It's basically like practice for being pregnant! I'll be a pro by the time the real thing comes!"

"Consider it marked." He smiled at me. "Now, do you need another ice pack? And can I shut off the camera yet?"

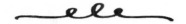

July 3 was intense. The side effects of the Lupron and birth control hit me hard. I had piercing cramps in one specific spot in my abdomen, which made it so I could hardly move. Luckily, it was a day off from work, so I could curl up on the shower floor, but it completely took my breath. They did the Lupron shots to prevent ovulation. Ovulation needed to occur only after meticulous monitoring and within a specific time frame. Because of this hormone cocktail, there was a laundry list of side effects that could hit you at any given time, and the nurses warned me of the list and cautioned me to avoid all things ibuprofen and stick with acetaminophen. I was an ibuprofen girl. It worked for me. So not being able to use it for the next however many months was going to be interesting. A small price to pay for a baby though, so I'd suck it up and do what I could. But it didn't mean that I couldn't lament while curled up on the bathroom floor, damning them all and trying to bargain with Josh to bring me some ibuprofen because it would work better.

Thankfully, he held fast against my pleas.

Once the wave of pain subsided, we had some errands to run in town, so we headed out to go shopping. Ten minutes after four o'clock, as we pulled into the parking lot of the sporting goods store, I got a phone call from the IVF Insurance coordinator at the clinic. She was calling with a quick update and said that she had just submitted my information for the cycle to insurance, and my carrier said (paraphrasing here), "uh, no. We don't have a referral for Ashley to go out of state for infertility treatments. Absolutely not. Hopefully, she hasn't started her cycle yet."

My heart started pounding, and I felt nauseous.

"What do you mean?!" My pitch flew off the handle at the end. I was panicking.

"You need to call your PCP immediately and have them get that referral to insurance. Also, you were supposed to have an important appointment tomorrow to change your Lupron dose, add in your other medications, Follistim and Menopur, and also complete the standard bloodwork/ultrasound. However, because your insurance provider didn't authorize the cycle, we can't do that anymore. If you were to come down anyway, then that's fine. We just need a payment of $8,000 tomorrow before we can do anything."

"What!?" I shrieked. Josh glared at the phone in my hand. My speakerphone kept him apprised of the latest bomb.

"Yes, but if you can get me the authorization number by the end of the day, you can continue with your appointment tomorrow as planned." She stated the steps that I would have to take and then ended it with, "so just let me know and have a great fourth of July."

Josh looked at me slowly. "Well, she clearly dropped the ball on submitting our cycle to insurance on time."

"And we're paying for it." I started to cry big, fat, snotty tears. He gathered me in his arms as much as he could from across the center console and snuggled into me. "What am I supposed to do?" I sobbed out. "I've already started taking the drugs. Tomorrow is a big appointment. I'm literally scheduled to have my tentative retrieval next weekend!" I wailed into his shirt.

"Okay, maybe we can fix this. She seemed eager to get off the phone, and it's four-twenty on the day before the fourth of July, but maybe we can fix this. Get your PCP on the line and see if we can expedite the referral to the insurance company and have her resubmit. Then, we can call back the IVF clinic and see if they have a copy on file. When the cross-border referral drama happened, you went through all these hoops with them a couple of weeks ago too, so they must have one on file. Maybe they can fax that to insurance. We got a plan. We just need to be speedy about it." He tried to rally the troops — me.

I hopped out of the truck, so I could pace on the median and called my PCPs office to see if I could get my referral faxed. The uncompromising lady on the phone must have been the same one from months prior because she gave me the same song and dance about how the referrals were handled out of house, and then she tried to hang up without letting me explain. I interrupted in time, saying that I already had one and that insurance had approved all the visits and drug prescriptions thus far for the IVF stuff, so the referral existed already. We just needed a copy faxed over again. She once again told me I needed to get a copy from the referral outsourcing center and hung up.

I wanted to blow a gasket, but I held it together long enough to call the number she gave me for the referral company. The figurative angel on earth that worked there promised to provide a reference number that I could give the insurance coordinator once I called her back. She also vowed to re-fax the referral to the insurance company.

I then called the insurance company, compulsively checking my watch as they placed me on hold after hold. Josh asked me as I paced back and forth and played the annoying On Hold music for us,

"Remember when the clinic contacted your insurance to ask about IVF, and your insurance said you weren't covered?"

Yes, dear. It was only a month ago." I wasn't in the mood for a walk down memory lane.

"Yeah, and do you remember calling them after the clinic called you and having another agent tell you that you were covered?"

I looked at him, unimpressed. "Yes?"

"Well, maybe the insurance company actually has the referral, and it's just misplaced, or someone doesn't know where to look."

"That's an optimistic way to look at it." There was a break in the music, and I shushed Josh frantically while I waited for someone to talk. But nope, just a lag in the music.

As he said something again, the music stuttered once more, and this time, someone started speaking!

I gave my personal information to confirm who I was; the seconds ticked by in my head, and I nervously waited to explain the situation to the agent who was plunking away on her keyboard. When I was done with my word vomit and took a breath, the lovely agent did her best to help.

"We have your authorization here on file. I'm looking at it right now. It doesn't look like the form has a start date. We can't accept it if it doesn't have a start date. You'll need to contact your provider to get a start date added and send it back to us."

The bureaucracy of the whole thing was even testing Saint Josh's patience. We were down to the wire here.

I called back the referral agency, hoping I'd receive the same woman as before, and got a voicemail.

Because, of course, I would.

It was ten minutes to five o'clock on the day before a holiday.

Obviously, everyone would be gone.

So Josh and I had a decision to make.

My heart felt like lead as we moved back into the truck and buckled up. Infertility and the associated depression and mood swings had hit me like a wrecking ball. I didn't even recognize who I was anymore. I never used to have such wild swings of emotion. But nowadays, everything always seems like the end of the world. Though, in this scenario, it wasn't the end of the world. Just the end of Eight. Thousand. Dollars.

Of which we did not have.

We sat there for a minute, collecting our thoughts.

As we drove home, empty-handed from our failed shopping trip, we didn't speak. Instead, we just sat with our thoughts, trying to figure out our next move.

Two steps forward, one step back.

Though, to be fair, we were moving forward. Slowly.

As we crossed town lines, a ringing blared out from my phone. I didn't recognize the number, but I picked up and nearly had a stroke.

At five minutes after five, on the day before a holiday, the lady at the referral company wanted to make sure we were okay, so she waited for my return call just in case something else popped up. She missed my call when she stepped away from her desk for a minute. When she got my voicemail, she stayed late, re-completed the authorization with a start date - per my voicemail, re-sent it to insurance and the IVF clinic, and called the insurance company to confirm. She gave me the authorization number to give to my IVF clinic and wished me all the best and good luck with my cycle. The woman was an absolute angel.

As soon as she hung up, I frantically called back every number I had on hand for the IVF clinic. I needed to get that authorization number to the coordinator no matter what, but at this point, it was ten minutes after five, and no one was answering.

I then pulled up my mail app and emailed it to every single person who I had exchanged emails with that worked at the clinic. Each nurse, doctor, and receptionist received this authorization number with the promise that even though it wasn't received before the end of the business day, I would still be there tomorrow morning and be expecting treatment as if they had. Unfortunately, the IVF coordinator never gave me her email, so I left it on her voicemail and prayed that one of the other people on the email chain would forward it to her.

"Can one thing in this whole damn process just go off without a hitch? Just one time? Can we just not have a drama with at least one of our procedures? Please?" Josh asked the universe.

"To be fair, we have most of this covered by insurance. That was a miracle in and of itself. So we should at least take a minute and appreciate that." I said in response.

"Pffft." My normally optimistic husband scoffed at me. Even the unflappable Josh could get frustrated when the stars aligned. I think he usually hid it for my sake, choosing to be the levelheaded one in the relationship, which I appreciated. But apparently, the excitement of today was just one straw too many for my trusty camel.

"Some days, you're the hammer. Some days you're the nail. We'll head down tomorrow and see what they say. Maybe it will be smooth sailing from here on out." I tried reassuring him, but my heart wasn't in it either. Recovering from it all, I was so tired and beaten. Plus, I hadn't even taken my Lupron shot for the night. Oh, joy.

"Yeah, let's see what tomorrow brings." He mumbled back, eyes on the road.

Nineteen

LUCKILY, WHEN WE SHOWED up first thing at seven-thirty that morning, the lab got me right in for bloodwork, and the ultrasound technician called me back shortly after. No one mentioned a single thing about the insurance/referral hiccup from last night. Everyone seemed perfectly happy with 'servicing' us, even though the insurance coordinator wasn't in the office to verify the authorization number.

As the tech was performing my internal ultrasound, she gave me the layout for the next week and a half. All ultrasounds would be internal, with a big ole wand shoved up my vagina. By the time this part of my life was over, I'd hardly notice anything in there. As she was explaining the pictures on the screen, the nurse came in and explained our steps for when we got home.

"We'll call you by the end of the day today with your bloodwork results. We're looking at your estrogen and progesterone levels to make sure they're acceptable. The good news is that everything looks good on the ultrasound, so as long as your blood work is good, you can lower your Lupron dose when you do your shots. Tonight you will go from ten ml to five ml per shot. Withdraw your Lupron syringes like you've been doing, but do not inject it. Instead, put the cap back on and put it to the side. Then open up your Follistim package. It should be in your refrigerator, right?" She hurriedly confirmed. We nodded in confirmation. "Okay, good. That would have been a problem." She let out a small laugh.

"Open up the zippered Follistim case and pull out the Follistim injection pen. Unscrew the pen cap so it splits into two, and then take the cylindrical vial of medication and insert it into the metal spiral in the pen's core. Then screw the pen back together, crank up the dial to the prescribed dosage of 150, and screw one of the needles onto the top of the pen. Next, you will inject that dose into the Menopur powder vial."

"When I was inventorying everything, we had liquid Menopur vials as well?"

"That is just a solution to mix the Menopur powder if needed. We're not doing that for your cycle."

"Okay," I nodded and motioned for her to continue.

"Once you've injected your Follistim into the Menopur bottle via the rubber stopper, you can remove the needle to the Follistim pen, discard it, and put the Follistim supplies away. Finally, pick your Lupron needle back up and inject the Lupron into the Menopur vial. Leave the needle inserted, flip the vial upside down, and suck everything back up again. The solution in that needle will now be a solution comprised of Lupron, Follistim, and Menopur. When injecting yourself, it will be about 20 units in the syringe."

"So we're making a drug cocktail?" Josh asked.

"I guess you could call it that. Of course, people do it differently, but we find this method effective, and it saves the patient a couple of pokes."

"Appreciate it," I mumbled.

"And you'll do this every night until the day we tell you to stop. You'll both start taking antibiotics twice a day starting tomorrow. It can't be taken with other medication or with dairy, though, so plan accordingly. Then it will be your Trigger Shot and then your Retrieval day! We'll monitor closely between now and then to ensure everything looks good."

"Sounds good!" I said. As the ultrasound tech cleaned off the ultrasound wand and rolled the cart out of the room, I nodded my head along as the nurse was speaking. Eager to have the next two weeks over with so we could know how many eggs we would get.

"Remember to call if there is any pain." She stressed to me. "And always give a shout if you have questions."

"You got it," I affirmed, twirling my thumbs idly. More than ready to go home, relax, and let my body start making some follicles.

We said our goodbyes and then made our way down to the lobby and out to the parking lot. As it was Independence Day and not even eight-thirty, the parking lot was near-empty. Josh and I looked at each other in relief once we finally got in my car and buckled our seatbelts.

"I can't believe they saw us and didn't ask about any of the insurance crap!" Josh laughed out.

"Maybe she made it sound like a bigger deal than it was?" I questioned.

"Who knows!" The relief in his voice was clear. "Who cares! As long as they saw us. I guess that's what matters."

I hummed my agreement and found a song on my phone to blast through the Bluetooth. As we pulled out of the parking lot, Josh leaned harder on the brakes.

"Stay straight, and we head home. Take a right... and we can grab some pancakes..." He suggested.

I smiled at him. "Right." I agreed.

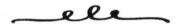

I gently placed my phone on the kitchen counter in front of me. I had just parked my car when I received a call from the now-familiar 413 number. The only calls I ever received from 413 were from our IVF clinic, so I was prepared for them to ask me to come in for a monitoring appointment or something of the like. Maybe something came up after looking at my ultrasound printouts from yesterday's appointment. I certainly didn't expect another insurance headache.

The insurance coordinator called to let me know that the authorization number we gave her on Monday was insufficient and that the insurance didn't fully approve our cycle. I literally could not help her any more than I already had. Each time I spoke with insurance, they told me I was covered, and my cycle was approved. I didn't know what was happening on her end and if it was related to the cross-border referral piece or what, but I asked her to call the insurance company again and talk to someone else because I was told on Monday that everything was approved and it was full-steam ahead.

We got off the phone with her, promising that she'd try a different agent, and two minutes later, I received the latest call from a 413 number, to which I begrudgingly answered. Another person from the IVF clinic informed me that the coordinator was on the phone with an insurance agent and trying to figure this out and that they'd let me know what they found out. I was unsure of the purpose of that call other than to stop me from downing a bottle of whiskey to wash away the dramatics of yet another IVF mishap. But as I wasn't a drinker, that must not have been the reason...

I went to the kitchen and grabbed some quick food for dinner. Josh had a soccer game after work today, and I had a softball game to get to, so I did my typical, low-maintenance thing–an instant breakfast mix with water and an English muffin with peanut butter. Boom. Quick and easy.

As I was eating my minimal-effort required dinner, I was scrolling through social media on my phone when a text binged across my banner screen. Our friends, who were doing infertility testing, Jamie and Chris, had received their referral to Burr Medical with us. As I was shooting texts back and forth with her and giving her my lowdown on the various road bumps so far, I couldn't help but feel excited. It's probably not good to feel excited that someone else might go through IVF, but it was a sense of solidarity and a relief that someone else was going through the same thing. She'd met the same doctors and nurses and had the same tests and headaches. We could commiserate, complain, and rejoice together. Plus, it was one step close for them as well, and as a person who was desperate for steps forward, I know the relief that comes with that knowledge.

I jogged up the stairs to grab my softball jersey and bag and was gone for all of three minutes. But by the time I returned to the kitchen, I had two missed calls from Josh. My husband isn't the type of person to call multiple times, so I immediately called him back.

"What's up?" I asked when he answered.

"Just wanted to let you know my boss caught me on the way out the door. I have to go to a customer in Arizona in August for a week. He said he knows we're in the middle of an IVF cycle right now, but it's pressing. Otherwise, we'd postpone it. He mentioned there is a little wiggle room. I could choose to go in the first or second week of August. But either way, I'm headed to Arizona during the first half of August."

"That's when we're supposed to be doing our transfer." I reminded him, trying to suppress the freak-out. I stalled as he spoke but realized that I needed to multi-task or I'd be late for the game. So I grabbed my stuff and held my phone to my ear as I locked up the house behind me.

"I know, dear. That's why I'm calling. I figure you probably had more information than me on when it's most likely to occur, so I wanted to check with you on which week was best."

Everything in me was trying to erupt into a panic, but the more rational part of me kept saying that this seemed like a manageable issue, so I subdued the urges and plowed on.

"I think we'll know more next week when we see how things are progressing. When do you need to give him an answer?"

"Sometime in the next couple of weeks. We don't need much notice."

"Well, that's good at least," I said as I pulled out of our driveway. As I did a head check on a blind corner coming off our road, I felt an uncomfortable twinge in my abdomen. I was already crampy and tired from having my period, but I definitely felt like the Lupron and the drug cocktail from last night possibly made things a little worse.

This would probably be my last week of softball. I was advised to stop playing next week before the retrieval because I would be swollen and bloated from the stimulation drugs. Basically, each follicle that I was growing would grow into the size of a grape. I didn't know how many my body would produce, but my imagination pictured a bushel of grapes massively expanding in my belly as they grew and grew before retrieval. Too many was a bad thing. Too few was a bad thing. My body needed to Goldilocks this bitch and get it 'just right.' I wasn't confident in my body's ability to do that anymore, so I braced for anything.

With the growth of the follicles, hopefully with healthy eggs inside, any twisting, like when you're up at bat, could cause fallopian torsion, and they could get all twisted, which could cause the loss of blood flow, which could lead to tissue death. All in all, it didn't sound good. So no softball next week.

Plus, after retrieval, I'd be swollen and tender, so no softball after retrieval either.

And then, after the transfer, I'd be carrying my life's most precious cargo and wouldn't want to cause any unnecessary jolts or bangs that could cause it to abort, so no softball then either. Not that the doctors said that. I said that. There's no way I could live with myself if the cycle worked, just to accidentally receive a line drive or pitch to the stomach and have it result in a miscarriage.

Nope. I couldn't mentally hack it. Plus, it was a pretty expensive procedure to risk if something went wrong. So I removed that risk factor.

In summary, pretty much no more softball after tonight.

After catching up on our days, informing him of the insurance update, and wishing each other good luck at our games, we said our goodbyes and hung up. We were both athletes, though we both had tremendously different attitudes towards sports.

Josh played to win. 100%. If you weren't going to win, then why bother playing?

I played to have fun. I played for the love of the sport. For teamwork, camaraderie, and the self-challenge. If I was part of a winning team-great. If we lost? Well, did I have fun playing? Then okay, it was all good. Some people on the softball team had Josh's outlook on the sport. I think I was one of the few outliers with my attitude, but I was used to that. Not many people shared my outlook. I played because I loved the sports I played. I didn't need to win. It was a bonus–who didn't love to win? And no, I don't like to lose. But I'm also not the type of person who brings the loss home with me. I wasn't going to dwell on it or get pissed after a game. I wasn't going to let it affect my attitude and outlook toward life because no one else should have to be poisoned by a bad attitude like that.

However, even though Josh played to win, I got lucky with my guy.

As competitive as he was, and that was very, he never brought it home. He was never sour after a game. By the time he got home, he had processed the loss and moved on. I appreciated that about him because I know he worked hard at mastering that over the years. And it made it much easier to know that we could lament and complain about bad calls after our games were done, but at the end of the day, they were out of our minds, and we'd be back to cuddling in bed watching our favorite shows in no time.

I like to think that infertility and the journey we had been on aided a bit in that perspective too.

Because whether it was a bad loss or a blown call-it wasn't infertility.

Twenty

DAY THIRTEEN OF MY cycle brought us back to Burr Medical for our first monitoring appointment after starting our Trifecta shot. The skin of my stomach on either side of my belly button was now slightly black and blue, with multiple pinpricks scattering the sides. The second insertion of the needle into the rubber stopper to pull up the Menopur and Follistim combo significantly dulled the needle. Therefore, the trifecta shots were pretty painful going in. Dart-like motions were necessary, and you needed to commit, or the needle would just bounce off your skin. At least, that's the way it was for me. The plunger was also slow to depress because the syringe would flex and bend under pressure too, so you had to apply some weight to the plunger to make it go. Combine those two things with some medication that burned *quite a bit*, and you got yourself an unpleasant shot experience. I developed a pneumonic remembering device to remember what side to poke myself on. If it was an even day (the second, fourth, sixth, fourteenth, etc.) of the month, then I injected myself on the left side because they both had E's. Otherwise, I'd inject on the odd side. Obviously, if one side was still particularly sore, I could bounce that schedule, but so far, it had worked well.

I had been taking Gonadotropins for five days now and was definitely starting to feel bloated and tired. Softball and golf the days before had been slightly uncomfortable with all of the twisting and pivoting. I wondered how coaching field hockey this fall would go if this cycle failed and I had to continue with this process. There was something to be said for a coach that could demonstrate the moves at speed versus one that had to do them in ginger slow motion... Yet another reason this cycle needed to work... For my coaching career... Right.

Josh and I woke up at five to start the long drive into Massachusetts. We arrived at the clinic a little after seven, logged into the IVF center upstairs, and dragged our feet back downstairs into the lab. Luckily things were quiet – given that it was a Sunday, so they got me in pretty quickly. I recognized several of the phlebotomists and made small talk with them as they tied my arm off and drew my blood. As we chatted, I mentioned that I'd be in a lot going forward for IVF monitoring, and I got a "Girlllll, damn. One of my girls did that and that shit ain't easy. You got this, Boo. I'll make a note in your file so that we'll use the tiny needles to keep your elbows healthy next time. You'll be in here a lot, so whatever we can do to help. I gotchu girl."

The interaction had me smiling while we walked back upstairs to the ultrasound rooms. As I took off my pants, hopped up on the bed, and draped the towel over my lap, I wondered to Josh how anyone could just "get used to this."

"I'm sure when you're having it done every other day, you become desensitized to it. And from what I understand, you won't care if the Queen of England walks in on you when you're in labor. You'll show her the family heirlooms without even blinking an eye."

I laughed, as he intended, and there was a soft knock on the door.

The ultrasound tech rolled her cart into the room and dimmed the lights. As she had me lean back, she advised me to tap my toes whenever I felt discomfort. Sometimes the wand needed to be pushed around a little bit to get a good look. She explained that if I tapped my toes in the stirrups, it might distract me enough from what was going on inside of me.

I didn't understand what she meant... until I did it.

Toes tapping slightly frantically, I eyeballed the ceiling and wondered how much longer she'd spend looking.

"Hmm." She said. That didn't sound like a good hmm.

"What is it?" My head shot up to look at the monitor.

"Well, you never really know what you're going to get, but you had a fairly unremarkable history and no PCOS. So it's surprising, but I only see one follicle growing on your right side. It measures at around a nine" She trailed off as she twisted the ultrasound wand again. This time I barely flinched. I was focused on the monitor and not on the pressure from the wand.

"Hmm. Okay, let's try the other side." The pressure reversed. Rather than feeling a stretch on the left side, I felt the wand rub on the right and push up into the left. My eyes stayed glued to the screen as I felt Josh's hand slide into mine on the table to my right. "Okay, that's much better. That's what I was expecting to see on the right. Here. Let's count..." As she moved the wand around, her other hand was doing all sorts of magic on the ultrasound ball and button keyboard in front of her. She took snapshots, quick measurements, and other notes without pausing. It was second nature to her, and she was a rock star.

The coordination alone impressed me, never mind the actual interpretation of the images.

"We have either nine or ten on this side. Not sure if I'm double counting that one or not. The biggest one is nine. The others are eights."

"Millimeters?' asked Josh.

There was a soft knock on the door, and Denise, another tech walked in.

"Yes," answered the ultrasound tech. She looked at Denise and recapped quickly. "One follicle on the right, nine or ten on the left. One follicle at a nine, the rest at eights."

"That's great!" Denise encouraged. She made notes on her notepad and sat next to the sink. She flipped through a couple of pages, shut the cover, and sat back. "Okay, that's great news. Don't worry about the right side. Sometimes one side just produces more than the other. I'm not going to adjust your dose. We'll keep you at the same levels and have you return on Wednesday for another round of bloodwork and ultrasound. If they grow according to what I'm expecting, they'll be measuring at twelve tomorrow, fourteen on Tuesday, and hopefully fifteen on Wednesday. Depending on your bloodwork and the sizes, we will look at your trigger shot on Wednesday or Thursday night, with retrieval on

Friday or Saturday morning!" She was pleased with these results, and her visible satisfaction bolstered my spirits. I was still a little salty with my right side for underperforming.

"Did you guys decide whether you were doing genetic screening or not? I know there was some discussion about it with Dr. Sadia, and we don't recommend the process for your case, but ultimately, it's your decision."

"Yes, we want to do PGS," Josh confirmed. She looked at him, nodded, and made a quick note on her notepad again.

"Ideally, we'll get a couple of follicles in the sixteen range during retrieval because ICSI likes the bigger ones. So hopefully, they'll continue this growth rate." Her face turned more serious. "However, even though you have ten follicles now, they might not all continue to grow. Some stop growing due to various reasons – nature is fickle. Additionally, going back to the orientation slides, only about 70% make it through the fertilization process. So 30% might not be viable after going through ICSI anyways. I just like to remind people of that. And I can see by your face right now." She said while eyeing me. "You're already looking at the negative. You've already been through so much to get here, and I totally get it. I need you to stay positive and know that you can't influence any of this; it only takes one to stick. One sticky little embryo, and you have your baby. Stay positive."

She made a few notes again and looked up, "Okay, no changes to your drugs, but do you have any questions?"

Josh and I had gone over our questions in the car on the drive down. "Yes, we have three." Josh started.

Denise was moving to stand up but settled back into her chair. "Okay, what do you have?"

"I want to talk about the schedule of," Josh started and was quickly interrupted.

She outlined, again, the timeline for the next two weeks with the retrieval, testing, results, and the future communication of those results to us. For about two minutes, we let her ramble on, answering a question that wasn't asked.

"Yeah... thank you. We got all that. I was actually wondering about the schedule for the transfer..."

He was once again interrupted as she answered what she thought our question was going to be.

Josh sighed softly next to me.

When she slowed down, he once again started back up to ask the question that she didn't let him ask.

"I have to travel for work. I'm trying to pick a time that won't interfere with the transfer; we wanted to know if you had a timeline for the expected transfer window so I can advise my boss on which week would be best?"

She blinked at him. "Well, that's all dependent on a lot of things we can't control. We can roughly count out three weeks with the PGS testing timeline and the need for a period cycle between the retrieval and the transfer, but we won't know until we're closer to that time. Is that all?" She moved to stand.

"No!" I rushed in to say. "What do we do on the day of the retrieval if Josh can't... you know... perform under pressure?"

"Don't get her wrong. I'm pretty sure I will not have a problem with that. I literally had to do it in a public bathroom at one point with a guy knocking on the door outside, so I'm not as worried about it as my dear wife is." Josh laughed.

"We have methods. Don't worry. You could always freeze a sample beforehand, but that's expensive and time-consuming. And you'll have better results with fresh sperm. We can always use electroshock therapy to remove the sperm as well." I quickly changed my level of degree of concern. Yeah, I'd trust that Josh had this covered...

She clapped her hands together quietly, "Okay, so if that's all..." And she stood up quickly and opened the door to usher us out.

"Actually, we had three questions." Josh and I continued to sit there.

It was a Sunday morning and all, but only one other couple was in the waiting room. So there was no reason for the rush out the door. But still, even though we had another question for her, she stood in the open doorway and paused to let me ask it.

"Umm, about Ovarian Hyper Stimulation Syndrome." I started. Not sure if it was protocol to ask medical questions with the door open. But I persevered and continued, "Can I drink water now, or will that fluid work against me after the retrieval? I don't want to have all this fluid in me that fills up the emptied follicles and gives me OHSS. I've read that it's pretty terrible."

She looked at me like I was insane. "OHSS happens after the retrieval. Not before. And you aren't a likely person to experience it as you only have ten follicles... the chance of you developing it is very unlikely. So yes you can drink as much water as you want. We recommend people stick to electrolyte-heavy drinks when they are likely to develop it after retrieval, but again, that's not you. Is that all?" Once again, she seemed like she had someplace to be.

I just accepted that that was as good of an answer as I would receive from her and nodded along, letting her off the hook. She closed the door behind her and vamoosed.

Josh was incensed. "What the fuck was that? She doesn't have the time to sit down and discuss something that her patient is concerned about?"

"It's fine. Let's just get out of here."

"It's not fine. You're going through a traumatizing experience. It's a Sunday fucking morning. I understand that no one wants to be here. We don't want to have to be here. But it's not like she had a waiting room full of people because it is a Sunday fucking, morning! So, really? She couldn't make sure that we, mainly you, were comfortable because she had to rush out to bring in the only other couple here. No, it is not okay what she did to you!"

"From what I've read, I'm not likely to develop it. Especially with my limited follicle numbers, so I can see why she'd dismiss the question."

"No, Ash. That's not okay, whether or not you've researched it. You're not here because this is a choice. This is our only option. So if you have something that's on your mind, with the amount of money that they're charging us and our insurance, during the most vulnerable part of our lives, they should make the time to answer your question, not rushing us away, or standing in the fucking door!"

Josh is the most even-tempered person I know. But when pushed over that edge, boy oh boy, watch out.

I started my tried-and-true diffusion tactic. Rambling. Ashley-style. "I wish I'd get OHSS." I mumbled as I stood up.

"What!" He whipped his head to look at me sharply.

"Well, I don't wish that I'd get it. Because... obviously... it sucks. And it is dangerous. But I wish I had the opportunity to get it. I wish that my body was reacting enough to the trifecta shot that I had tons of follicles, and there wasn't a concern that we were doing all of this just to end up with one or no embryos. So, I misspoke. I don't wish that I'd get it. I just wish that my body was producing as it should. Heck, when we came for our baseline appointment last month, I had seven on the right and eight on the left. I assumed that once I was on the stimulation cocktail, I'd be popping up follicles left and right and have tons to work with. But instead... this is what we're working with."

He looked at me, and his expression softened.

"Worth every heartache?"

"Worth every heartache," I confirmed as we exited the building.   ***

"Hi, I have a retrieval this weekend, and my husband and I each have to take two pills of Doxycycline per day. I just counted the pills this morning before leaving for work, and we don't have enough to bring us to this weekend. I need to place a refill stat, please."

I panicked this morning when I realized that we were short on antibiotics, so I tried to call the pharmacy as soon as they opened.

I had tried calling the IVF clinic already to ask if it was a big deal or not, but couldn't get ahold of the IVF nurses that could answer that question. The receptionist took a message for me and said they'd be in touch. I also couldn't afford to wait for a phone call and miss a day or two of antibiotics due to a delay in processing and delivery, so I figured I'd be proactive and order now, and if I didn't need them, then okay. Better safe than sorry.

I went about my normal workday, finishing up extensions and doing some prep work for some audits that were coming up. I had several June 30 year-end clients that needed to be sent engagement letters as well as their annual document request list for their audits. Luckily the lists were mostly the same from year to year, so I was able to listen to some IVF podcasts while updating the lists.

I received a call from the IVF clinic at one point in the afternoon but was in a meeting and couldn't answer. I returned to my office to hear a relatively snippy voicemail from Denise.

"Ashley, I see a note here saying that you had a question about your drugs. We just saw you yesterday. I told you there were no changes in your drugs or doses. Please don't change anything and continue to administer as you were prescribed. I told you that we'd call you if there was anything different that you needed to do."

Immediately, I felt frustrated that she was getting bitchy with me, but redirected my frustration and realized that my message was probably delivered incorrectly. It sounded like I was indeed asking about my prescription doses rather than my prescription of antibiotics. I could understand why she'd sound frustrated and fed up with having to return the phone call. Regardless, she didn't answer my question. I'd have to call back and confirm my real question with her once I got into my car.

After I got a hold of them and clarified my question, the nurse seemed less pissy. She informed me that I only needed seven days of antibiotics and that I didn't need to place a rush order for more. Drats. Oh well. I was partially frustrated because after she was so impatient with us yesterday, she was now impatient on the phone and with her answers too.

The hormones were starting to take their toll. I felt nauseous, swollen, crampy, and exhausted. My midsection felt full and tender. There was a constant cramp pulsing on my left side; nothing super intense, but always there. My lower back on the left side was uncomfortable as well. I just felt off. And the needles were really giving me issues at night when I did the shots. It wasn't quite a 'slide in like warm butter' experience. There was absolute resistance on the needle tip when I'd insert it. Some nights, I'd have to give it an extra bit of force to get it in my belly. Those nights were painful. Then, the injection itself burned going in. Josh and I developed a good routine where we'd set up the camera and record a video about the symptoms and drama of the day while mixing the drug cocktail. Then we'd record ourselves doing the shot. Some nights were relatively quick. Some nights showed me swearing like a trucker because it was so painful. I liked that we were recording the videos though. I thought we'd look back on these videos one day and be grateful that we documented the process and dramas as well as we did.

I felt relatively okay until this point but was really starting to feel the effects of the hormones. I was beginning to regret that we were doing PGS testing because I was starting to get tired of all this back and forth and just wanted to get things done and over with. PGS testing required an additional month between the retrieval and transfer, so more waiting was scheduled on the docket. Additionally, not only was my stomach full and crampy, but the skin of my stomach on either side of my belly button was tender and bruised. I entertained the idea of switching to a different injection site, but I didn't want to mix it up and ruin any established tradition. As a softball player, I was big on superstitions. Regardless of my beliefs though, I had to admit that I was losing steam with the current shot locations. With my exhaustion and highly emotional state, I might have to risk the wrath of the superstitious fates and try something new to give my poor belly a break. Even just for a night.

Josh and I used a catchphrase whenever I was feeling overwhelmed. When the shots didn't go in easy or were particularly painful, we'd remind each other, "worth every shot." When an invoice was much higher than we expected, we'd remind each other, "worth every penny." And when something went wrong or not according to my master plan, we'd remind each other, "worth every heartache."

We had been saying those phrases a lot lately.

Wednesday finally arrived, and we drove down for our seven o'clock arrival time.

True to her word, the nice phlebotomists hooked me up with the thinnest needles, but it didn't help that much. At this point, my elbow was scabbed, bruised, and tender. My other elbow didn't have a vein that would work, so it was the same one-centimeter range they pulled blood from on my right elbow, and that shit was getting old.

But there was good news during the ultrasound. The right-side follicle was now at a sixteen-point five - which was awesome. The ultrasound tech asked me if I had any symptoms when she was scanning the left side.

I was all too eager to discuss my suffering of the last few days, and she chuckled with understanding.

"Yes. I can see that. Your left side is over-compensating a bit. You're very full over here. I see one at seventeen, a couple at sixteen, one or two at fifteen. And I have another at thirteen. So yes, you will feel uncomfortable and like your stomach is full of swollen organs."

Ding ding ding.

So at least my symptoms were expected.

"We'll call you with your bloodwork results later, but you'll probably be taking the trigger shot tomorrow and not tonight to give the smaller follicles a chance to grow a bit more. This means you'll be looking at a Saturday retrieval date. But we'll confirm with you later."

As we were driving home, I was hit with a wave of exhaustion. Not for sleep. But just of this process is navigating work schedules and taking time off to attend appointments. I told myself that it was worth it all but was it really? The pain during the shots. The pain during the blood draws—the internal ultrasounds. The hormones were making me wonky and cranky. Not to mention the general worry that I was experiencing daily. This morning was a perfect example. If we postponed the trigger shot until tomorrow so the smaller follicles could grow, were we damaging the bigger follicles? Could they burst? Could they die? Could a follicle get too big? Were we sacrificing the current large ones with the hopes the smaller ones would achieve the right size? I had no idea, but I was sick of asking questions. I was sick of *needing* to ask questions. Particularly I was getting sick of having these questions, not receiving good answers, and then being asked by my mom or friends the same questions that I was wondering. It just brought up the fact that I didn't know. I didn't know *anything* during the *whole* process. My mom was very invested in our progression. She wanted to know how I was doing, along with any updates. She was my mom. Besides Josh, she was my best friend. But her frequent questions about stuff I didn't know, or stuff I decided I couldn't spend my time worrying about, was a constant reminder that I was at the mercy of medical professionals that didn't always give me the time of day. I wasn't always nice. I'd let my frustrations boil over and answer impatiently. I was just so...

tired. Just plain tired and very ready for this IVF business to be over so we could move on to the next phase of our life. Desperately I hoped that we wouldn't have to do this again.

Our phone call with the nurse that afternoon was quick. Dr. Sadie had reviewed my results of everything from that morning and ordered me to continue with my prescribed shots tonight, as discussed earlier. The nurse told me I was at risk of developing OHSS after the procedure, which a part of me found slightly comical given that the other nurse had poo-pooed the question when I asked. Now, here I was, being told I could develop it with my handful of follicles.

She reminded us that my retrieval would be exactly thirty-six hours after my trigger shot, which should be taken at seven-thirty the following night. I'd have a five-minute window to take the shot. She repeated this again very slowly to me and with great emphasis, causing my heart to start palpitating with the various what-if scenarios of what could go wrong.

What if the needle snapped and broke?

What if I got in a car crash on the way home?

What if Josh got hung up at work and couldn't make it home in time?

What if a meteor hit the continental US?

What if, after all of this, IVF still didn't work?

What if we never were able to have kids?

Crazy person – that's me.

Therefore, shots as usual that night to give one more day of growth to my follicles. Then, the trigger shot of pure hCG tomorrow night to force ovulation. Thirty-six hours later, I'd have my retrieval surgery to remove the follicles.

We were making progress, and I prayed it would be worth every bit of the heartache, pain, and wait.

Twenty-One

"I'm so thirsty." I groused to Josh for the hundredth time that morning. He rolled his eyes and continued to play on a brain app on his phone.

They instructed me not to drink water after nine last night, and I felt it. I couldn't even sip a teeny bit of water after brushing my teeth. I was parched. They made it seem like the absolute end of the world if I consumed even an extra drop of water before the surgery, and with something this important, I wasn't leaving room for interpretation or any 'guidelines rather than actual rules' riff-raff. Josh thought a sip of water wouldn't kill anyone. But he wasn't a medical professional, so I wasn't letting my dear husband or Dr. Google influence me. No peer pressure for me. And no water for me.

No siree.

Not with something this valuable.

So here we were. Saturday morning with a six-thirty arrival time. Which meant we left our house at five. Which means I was up at four-thirty.

You can imagine how great I slept the night before. Not nervous or excited at all... The trigger shot went surprisingly well. At seven-thirty on the dot, Josh injected me. I picked the least sore, bruised, and callused spot on my stomach, hoping that it wouldn't be as tender when this next medication went in. I pinched a small chunk of fat and skin, leaned back in my chair, braced my feet, and gave Josh his cue on when to thrust in the needle. We had already been through this song and dance sixteen times, as it was day seventeen of shots. As I was doing my preliminary exhale before the big exhale, Josh injected me early. He expected my customary panic on the count of 'two' of the "one, two, three" and jumped the gun so I wouldn't call it off and have us restart again.

My mom and dad were over to cheer us on. When we were done, my mom's underwhelmed exclamation of "that was it!?" had me laughing off any residual pain from the pinch of the needle. Though, to be fair, the Trigger Shot needle was crisp and went in like my belly was room temperature butter. If only my other needles had been so sharp up to this point. I think my belly would be a lot less bruised.

We had a bit of a false alarm yesterday (par for the course, really) when a nurse called me and reminded me I was to take my trigger shot that night at seven-thirty. I think my heart might have stopped for a second or two. Then, I panicked and asked, "no... wasn't that supposed to be last night?" She frantically started shuffling papers around, and I heard her breathe a sigh of relief into the phone.

"Oh, okay. Yes, I see. You're right–the trigger was supposed to be last night..."

"Yes," I breathed. Now a little annoyed. Why couldn't they remember anything about my case? Why was every conversation with one of them a revelation? I felt like every single time I spoke with a nurse there, they didn't know who they were talking to and were just reading a standard script to me, then I'd have to remind them about something, and they'd say, "Oh, yeah. Then just keep doing that..."

It was an understatement to say I was less than impressed with their attention to detail.

So there I was, dehydrated and stinky. Stinky, because they said not to use any deodorant, nail polish, hair products, etc., in the hours before the procedure because it could affect the eggs during retrieval. So even though I wasn't stinky, I still felt 'unclean.'

After we checked in at the IVF surgery window, they routed us into a back area with a surprising number of locks and antechambers. I don't know if many people tried to break into the IVF surgery center, but it was a Fort Knox compared to other hospitals.

The back area had four different bays with curtains for privacy. We were the first ones there and set up shop in Bay One. I was told to undress, don the hospital johnny, and get comfortable. The unknown nurse came back periodically for some easy chitchat and to share our excitement. As Josh and I sat there in nervous anticipation, I couldn't stop thinking that this was it. This was the start of our life. This was the moment that everything would begin. I couldn't wait to see how many eggs would be retrieved from my follicles. I couldn't wait to see the results of the PGS testing. I was already planning out ways to appropriately ask them to transfer the female embryo next month because I wanted a daughter first. As we waited, I schemed all of this out to Josh while he indulgently rolled his eyes at me and let me ramble. He agreed with my desire for PGS testing because he also felt that it would be a shame to do all of this only to transfer an incomplete embryo that wouldn't stick and develop. He didn't care about the sex of the resulting embryos, but I viewed it as a nice little bonus feature of the testing. The nurses had already warned me I couldn't select the sex of the embryo to be transferred when it was transfer time unless there were legitimate reasons, but I figured it couldn't hurt. My theory was that if I requested the female embryo because of male factor infertility and the cysts that could be genetic, they might view that as an acceptable request.

We'd see!

For shits and giggles, I peed on a pregnancy test and an ovulation predictor kit the prior night in a desire to see a positive test at least once in my life in case the IVF process went south. It was a waste of a test, but it made us laugh, and at that point, my nerves were so hyped up and on edge that the small chuckle from seeing a positive pregnancy test next to a positive ovulation test felt like a breath of fresh air. Josh also had a good laugh at me cradling my boobs all night long, as the boob pain had intensified tenfold since taking the trigger shot. As I sat in my hospital johnny waiting for them to roll me into the surgery room, I gingerly held my bra-free boobs and wished for a warmer blanket...

When a team of nurses and my doctor opened the curtain to ask if I was ready, Josh jumped up and kissed me goodbye. I squeezed his hand as they rolled my bed down the hall and looked at him as we approached the double doors leading to the surgery room.

"See you on the other side!" I couldn't stop smiling.

He bent down and kissed my forehead again. "See you soon!"

They pushed me through the double doors that could stop a missile, into a sterile operating room. The enormous bright lights on the ceiling instantly had me blinking and looking away. Soft music played in the background and a bunch of nurses bustled around.

A couple of nurses next to the operating table were arguing about which anesthesiologist was on duty that day.

"No, no, Dr. so-and-so is on today." One said while adjusting some tools on the table in front of him.

"No, he's not here. Your *favorite* is coming down to cover."

"But he's not scheduled."

"I know." The nurse opened his eyes dramatically. "This should be fun to watch."

So. That gave me warm fuzzies... Not.

I've seen my fair share of hospital shows. I didn't want to die on the table because the anesthesiologist was pissed he was working an unexpected caseload and forgot to dial back my anesthesia or something equally ridiculous.

I could only hope that my imagination was running wild and that the hospital shows were inaccurate. They were probably inaccurate.

Right?

Right.

Things moved fast from there. They positioned me on a table that gave me major Jesus and his Crucifixion vibes. My arms were extended out on little side tables out from the main table. More medical professionals entered the room and gave me an IV in my hand. I had to confirm my name and date of birth one more time and was told to rest my hand on the table with my palm facing up. My fear of IVs had not diminished during the IVF process, so the thought of resting my hand with an IV in it on the table made me want to vomit. That thought was quickly overridden by a slight uptick in fear when the anesthesiologist came in and told me I would feel some pain in my arm.

"I'm going to inject a medicine into your IV, and it's going to be uncomfortable. It will be intense, but it will only last about twenty seconds. Then we'll get a mask on you, and it will be time for a nap."

He didn't smell like alcohol or seem upset, so I felt like I was in excellent hands. I didn't feel the need to voice my Grey's Anatomy concerns.

As I gave my consent, one nurse popped over by my head. They added softly, "some people find that squeezing their hand open and shut helps."

I had no idea what he was talking about... until I did.

A wave of fire erupted in my hand. I looked over at it, expecting it to be in flames. The anesthesiologist murmured something to me I couldn't hear. The pain moved up to my elbow, and I started fidgeting slightly. I opened and closed my fist again and again. I started breathing heavier. I could hear the heart rate monitor beeps pick up. Suddenly, the room didn't feel so chilly. The pain intensified and moved up into my bicep. I started frantically opening and closing my first and tried to control my rapid breathing.

Good God. What was I doing here? First the HSG pain, and now this? Clearly, I couldn't handle this. Clearly, my body was not supposed to get pregnant. There's no way I could handle childbirth. Not if these minor procedures brought this amount of pain. Maybe my pain receptors were broken. Maybe my calibration when I was in the womb was screwed up, and I felt pain more intensely than others. I certainly wouldn't describe this as 'uncomfortable.'

"Eighteen, nineteen, twenty." The anesthesiologist finished.

And just like that, the pain dissipated.

Okay, phew.

A light sheen of sweat dotted my brow, and I berated myself for being such a pansy. It was just twenty seconds.

God, I was such a wimp (still am actually)!

My assigned IVF doctor made her way up to where my head was and asked some last questions. Then, with a big smile, she asked if I was ready.

As they put the mask over my face, I breathed a sigh of relief and started my nap.

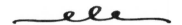

I woke up crying and apparently, it wasn't the first time. Josh had had the same conversation with me several times by now, and each time my memory would reset and start all over again.

I was a regular Adam Sandler rom-com.

I had told our wonderful nurse about my eye surgery... multiple times.

I also told her about PGS testing...multiple times.

I vocally thought through and developed a phone app that was linked to the embryologists' lab here at Burr Medical that would allow IVF patients to check on the status of their embryos throughout the incubation and fertilization process.

Apparently, I got hung up on what we would name it each time, end scene as I was brainstorming, and then repeat.

So I woke up crying. Again.

"I just feel so emotional right now!" I cried to Josh.

He patted my hand consolingly, but the man never put down his camera. He was determined to catch me in all my high glory.

As I tried not to rub my eyes and battle through the fog, someone from the embryology lab came in and gave the results.

"We retrieved ten eggs, which is great because we were only expecting nine!" I mumbled to her as I battled the brain haze and accidentally repeated myself yet another time. The lady was a saint for answering each time.

"Your husband gave us his sample while you were under, so we'll perform the ICSI procedure in four hours. Tomorrow morning, we'll check to see which ones are fertilized and then call you with the results. From there, we'll contact you on Day Three, which is Tuesday, with a status update, and then again on Day Five or Day Six.

I tried to understand what she was saying, but the world would never know why she tried speaking to a woman as she was coming out of anesthesia.

I asked her to repeat it a few more times until Josh took pity on her and released her from my memory loop that had become that poor nurse's prison. He confirmed he understood what she was saying and that she could go. He'd tell me what I needed to know again later.

After she left, I had a bit of a better memory recollection, and things started returning to me. I was feeling tentatively optimistic with the ten eggs. Typically, they advised a 40% attrition rate from retrieval through Day Five or Six, so we were looking at four viable embryos we could eventually transfer. Josh and I were tentatively thinking we'd have either two or four kids anyway, so it would be perfect if everything went according to plan.

But as I learned throughout this entire process. Life seldom ever goes according to plan.

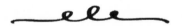

My pain started increasing almost as soon as I sat in the car to drive home. I had a cool outlet in my car that let us plug things into that I had never actually used, but I had read online that a heating pad would be my friend after the egg retrieval, so I brought one just in case. Almost immediately, I had that puppy plugged in and pressed up to my cramping belly. The doctors gave me a prescription for some strong pain meds that Josh and I had to swing by to pick up on the way home, but after an hour and a half in the car, my pain was significant enough that I just wanted to curl up in bed. So Josh first dropped me off at home and headed out to grab the meds.

As the day progressed, I tried to nap but was just so incredibly uncomfortable. It felt like my stomach had filled with water after the surgery, and it was making it hard to breathe. I couldn't lay flat without suffering from pain, nausea, and intense rib and collarbone pain, so I ended up crashing on the recliner to stay more inclined. In the morning, when I woke up, my entire body hurt. I also spent the whole night fighting the hot sweats. I stepped on the scale and I found I had gained five pounds. My stomach was incredibly swollen and puffy, and looked like I was six months pregnant. It was intense.

One of the IVF doctors called to ask how I was feeling and I listed my woes.

"Yeah, some people feel pretty sore after the retrieval, especially if they react funny to anesthesia. That's common. You have the list of things to look out for and know when to call us or when to head to the ER, correct?"

"Yeah, we have it on the counter." I rolled my eyes at Josh.

"Good. And you're not doing a fresh transfer because you're doing PGS, correct?"

"Right."

"If you have any Lupron left, just continue to take that. That can help regulate your hormones a little faster. As long as we aren't doing a transfer this cycle, just use up whatever Lupron you have left."

I gave a sobbing face to Josh as he watched me talk to her on speakerphone. He smiled and mouthed, "we're going in the butt finally!"

He kept trying to give me shots in my butt, thinking it would hurt less, but I wasn't convinced. Considering how my stomach was feeling now, I very well might let him inject me in the butt cheek so he could stay far away from my tender belly.

And god. My collarbones felt like they were hammered with a sledgehammer. They felt shattered.

Josh felt I was being overly dramatic with my descriptive complaints, but I felt they were right on the money.

God, how I hoped this would be the only retrieval we needed.

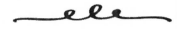

We had pretty good news on Tuesday when they called us with our Day 3 results. Seven of the ten eggs were fertilized. The nurse emphasized that they looked healthy and that all had eight cells apiece. Which, she explained, was a wonderful thing. I wasn't having the rib and collarbone pain anymore, but I had developed a slight pressure right in my sternum that made breathing hard. Bending over at night for the Lupron shots in the butt was becoming difficult. Not because of the pain but because of the increased difficulty breathing when bent over the table. I found that dropping 'trow' and bending over the table gave Josh a perfect canvas to choose the ideal place to inject me. I have much more junk in the trunk, if you know what I mean, so finding a non-bruised part was much easier than finding a spot in my belly.

I was semi-guilted into going to work on Tuesday by my boss, but by noon I was walking around like a neanderthal and couldn't stand upright, and my abdomen was swollen and tender. My normal pants wouldn't fit, and it just hurt to move. I huffed and moaned slightly whenever I had to move, and pivoting at the hips was impossible. At one point, one of my co-workers stopped and asked me if I was okay. Because I had told no one at work (besides my bosses) we were doing IVF yet, they didn't understand what was going on, and I'm sure I looked as awful as I felt. I ended up calling it a day at noon, went home, took some wonderful pain meds, and tried to ignore the pain screaming in my abdomen.

Thursday was more good news. Out of the seven, six had continued to grow. We saw a small decline from the original ten, but as 40% was the survival rate's target number, I felt pretty good about our results. We were still operating under the assumption that Josh was the main infertility cause, though I still wasn't 100% buying it. My cycles were too irregular and whacky not to have any responsibility for this unfortunate journey. It was probably just a mental thing, an irrational worry, but it would ping around in my head when I started feeling pessimistic about our chances. I beat those thoughts back with an ugly stick and tried to stay positive.

Six out of ten. Not bad.

The doctor said they weren't ready for biopsy yet, so they'd recheck them tomorrow and see if they were ready then. She mentioned in passing that biopsying the embryos sometimes acted as assisted hatching when transferring the frozen embryos. I thought that was interesting and found it encouraging that it might be a sort of 'leg up' for the embryos upon transfer. My breathing difficulties had only increased since Tuesday, and when I told the IVF doctor how I was feeling, she didn't seem surprised. She said that patients typically start to feel the effects of the trigger shot on Day 7–so I was on track for an exciting weekend. It had me counting my remaining pain pills and mentally bracing for the possible storm.

Worth every shot. Worth every heartache. Worth every penny. I just kept repeating it to myself.

Again.

And again.

And again.

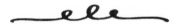

OHSS hit me like a ton of bricks on Friday morning. I called the clinic in a slight panic, barely able to breathe. I could hardly move and felt terrible. Josh was already at work, so I called my mom and asked her to drive down to the clinic with me. I hijacked her whole morning just so she could sit in a car for three hours and a waiting room for another one. Like a champ she never complained. They ran bloodwork and an ultrasound on me, but the fluid level wasn't high enough that they needed to drain me or anything. The ultrasound tech and doctor explained that my ovaries looked great, but when you have OHSS, the fluid sinks in your abdomen… because… you know… gravity. Since the bottom part of your abdomen is filled with water, it pushes all your other organs up. So basically, my organs were pushing up against my diaphragm and lungs, and that's what is causing all the pressure. It was interesting to imagine but painful to experience.

They encouraged more drinking and rest and said they'd call me later with bloodwork results. I wasn't experiencing a bad enough case to require drainage. Thank God.

When they called later that day with my bloodwork results, I was still feeling awful and highly emotional. I started calling that emotion 'trigger happy.' It was a little on-the-nose, but I felt it was accurate. It wasn't taking much to set me off in either direction, and I was unpredictable and unstable. When she said I had good bloodwork results, just some mild OHSS, I wanted to snap, 'if this is mild, what is severe?' but held my tongue. When she asked if I had heard from the lab about our embryos yet, she was surprised that hadn't. She put me on hold and checked for me.

And there it was.

The news that my Negative-Nancy-self had been expecting this whole time.

Two more embryos had 'died' overnight, and now we were down to four.

Josh pointed out that on the plus side, the PGS testing place would only test a certain number of embryos, and now we were certainly below the threshold. But even he couldn't shake the nerves that accompanied the news.

Four. Four chances. We wanted four kids. What were the odds that each one would successfully transfer and 'stick'? Not likely. So, if we really wanted four kids, then we'd likely have to do another retrieval because odds were, not all these little embryos would successfully turn into cute little babies.

As the news settled in, my mind started spiraling down that negative path. All the bad thoughts I had tried to keep at bay started piling up. I started wondering if I needed to refresh myself on the adoption research again. And then I chastised myself for treating adoption as a backup plan. Therefore, guilt was added to the mix of fun emotions. While all these toxic thoughts were running wild, I remembered just how awful and uncomfortable I felt.

"Maybe... we're not supposed to have kids?" I cried out brokenly to Josh, and he rubbed my back.

We were sitting next to each other on the love seat—my new sleep location for the past few days as I couldn't lay down without feeling like I was suffocating.

"Ash. We're meant to be parents. We were expecting this. Take a breath."

I tried to regulate my breathing more, but the OHSS made it even harder to cry properly. The realization made me feel even more miserable, so I just continued to cry brokenly.

"But look at the signs! Every step of the way, we've been met with roadblock after roadblock. It's unrelenting. I feel like God is trying to give us a sign."

"Ash. No. It's the other way around. Every step of the way, we've been met with a roadblock, and we've rallied and pushed forward every time. This is a life lesson—a character-building experience. We're learning about perspective. And I doubt God, if there is one, cares whether we have kids. But *we* care. And we'll be damn good parents." I was a believer in God; my husband was more on the Agnostic side of things. Neither one of us pressured the others. It may be odd, but it worked. "We're going to have kids. One way or another. Try to stay positive." He kept rubbing my back and was patting it emphatically every time he ended a sentence.

"These remaining four are like four remaining Spartan warriors. The other ones wouldn't have been able to stick. But these ones. These ones are fighters. These ones are helping Leonidas during the battle."

"Well, that ends poorly for them," I mumbled half-heartedly, but understood his point, and gave him a small smile.

I settled my breathing enough that I wasn't in pain every time I tried to suck in a breath, but now I just felt... unfinished. Like I had a big cry just waiting in the wings. Ready to burst out of me at the sight of a sad commercial, song, or memory. I was teetering on the edge but had staved it off for now. We'd see how long it would last.

Apparently, just until my shot that night...

Josh hit a tender spot in my butt cheek with the needle of the remaining Lupron, and it was the nail in the coffin. I went off the rails...The straw that broke the camel's back... Insert more colloquialisms here. I had them all.

After fifteen minutes of massive sobbing, I felt better. Less suffocated. Less suppressed. I had mentally (and physically) processed and took that time to rally the troops. We knew our next steps involved the subsequent round of drugs to prepare us for the frozen transfer cycle.

We just had to wait until my period started, and then we'd be on to the next phase of this journey.

Perseverance was my middle name.

Twenty-Two

"WE'RE ALREADY TWO AND half years into this thing, and having an embryo abort on us two months into a pregnancy because it had chromosomal abnormalities that we could have checked for but didn't would be..."

"Devastating." Josh finished my sentence succinctly.

"Exactly." I gave him a quick smile and looked back at the nurse. "So, yes, I know we didn't need to do PGS testing, but we'd rather have spent the money to confirm we were transferring healthy embryos rather than risk transferring one that was just going to abort on us later. Mentally, we've decided we don't want to handle that." I explained this for the fifteenth time to another nurse who had questioned why we'd want to do PGS testing when we're in our late twenties with no genetic markers in our history that would suggest a problem. After she gave me a loaded, "Okay then, I guess," and left, I looked over to Josh, and he rolled his eyes. We were interrogated about this decision several times now, and each time we had to explain our reasoning. It was getting old. The testing was done. The four embryos were all healthy. The invoice was already on our credit card.

I asked the doctor this morning what the genders of each of our four embryos were, and she got all huffy with me. Josh, ever the diplomat, diffused the situation, which I appreciated.

"We know we can't select which embryo is transferred. That's not why we're asking. We just want to know the sexes of them." I'm totally an empowered woman and all that, but I can't deny that when a man is direct, they get answers a lot easier than females because we were told that we had three boys and one girl frozen, ready to be transferred.

They wrote on a small paper what sex the one they were transferring today was, and they put it at the front desk. She sealed it and said I could open it after I left. I couldn't wait! I secretly hoped it was the girl.

"Speaking of PGS, if this cycle doesn't stick, do we want to do another retrieval to send to the PGS testing site, given that we've already paid for the testing of eight embryos, and they've only tested four?"

Josh took a minute to respond. His eyebrows scrunched together as he mentally thought through my proposal. He was sitting in the chair next to my gurney in hospital scrubs with a hairnet. He was able to come into the transfer room with me and watch the little embryo be inserted, but needed to be sterile. So once again, no deodorant, perfumes, or nail polishes for me. But this time, Josh had to be chemical-free as well. They gave me some meds to take about forty minutes before my appointment to help 'relax' me for the transfer. I thought that the first pill would be enough, so I didn't take the second. I still felt wired when we pulled into the parking lot thirty minutes later, so I popped the second just to finish mellowing me out.

Hence the very calm discussion about doing the awful egg retrieval again like it was no big thing.

"You bring up a good point," Josh slowly started, still visibly analyzing in his head. "We've already paid for those testing slots, and if this cycle isn't successful, it makes you wonder how successful the other attempts will be. We only have those testing slots for a year. So if you got pregnant, then no big deal. We're out that money anyway. It's a sunk cost. But if you don't get pregnant, then we'll have to do another retrieval anyway to get four kids... It's worth discussing further." He pinched his lips to the side and continued looking at a far spot across the room while thinking it over and speaking to me. You could tell he was distracted by the way he gazed off while thinking about it, trying to see all the sides of the, what I thought, simple proposal.

"And we have a lot of leftover drugs," I added, somewhat unnecessarily. "So we wouldn't have that much more in pharmacy costs."

"Yeah, they sent us a lot..." He agreed quietly, keeping in mind the other IVF patients in the rooms next to us.

"Would we want to deal with this whole retrieval process all over again years down the road when we'd potentially have a toddler at home? The back-and-forth and monitoring appointments with a baby would be tough, so maybe we get all the retrievals done now, so we're not having me deal with this recovery while chasing after a toddler?" The drugs were really working because the thought of another retrieval wasn't terrifying me as much as it would have a day ago.

"Yeah, something to think about."

"Just throwing it out there for later," I mumbled as I cozied deeper into my hospital bed, getting ready for a quick power nap before the transfer.

The prep work leading up to this moment to prepare my uterus for this transfer was relatively uneventful. After waiting and waiting and waiting for my period to start when the OHSS subsided and yielded no results, I jumped on the trusty dusty message boards and infertility forums and discovered that Lupron could be used to suppress periods. The doctor had told me to continue to take it until I used the bottle up, and it was accidentally postponing my period. After checking in with the clinic and confirming I could indeed stop the shots, I rejoiced, and we partied like it was 1999. Actually, no, we didn't. Josh fell asleep in bed watching wrestling and I read a book. But in my heart, I was partying because my butt didn't need a shot that night for the first time in thirty days.

Sure enough, the next morning, I started my period. Either very coincidental timing or my body really wanted to have a period, and the Lupron just kept shouting 'No!'

Josh laughed when I called him at work with an update. "It's only fitting that it took so long to start your period. It's almost karma. You had a period for four weeks straight a couple of months ago, and now here you are, wishing your period would have come sooner."

He wasn't wrong.

And that first period after the retrieval was a doozy. Blood clots galore. TMI, I'm sure. I usually felt like crap, but the plus side was no more shots! I only had to incrementally use the estrogen patches that they shipped me with the rest of our drugs and eventually added progesterone suppositories as well. I wasn't a big fan of those. More graphic information to be shared, but those suppositories go up your vagina.... And make a mess. I'm not a fan.

Then there was an insurance snafu–yes, another one–where the pharmacy said that I was only allowed one box of eight estrogen patches every twenty-eight days, and my copay for those would be $10. But, if I needed additional boxes within that time frame, I would have to pay $80 per box. My estrogen schedule had me changing one patch every two days, then two patches every two days, and then four patches every two days for up to three months after a positive pregnancy test. That $80 copay business would not fly. So that was a bit of an adventure I had to deal with when Josh was on his fated work trip. But onwards and upwards.

We were finally here.

August 16.

The day Josh and I might finally become parents.

In a true Schrödinger's box scenario, we would be both pregnant and not pregnant when we left for the day. For nine days after transfer, we wouldn't officially know whether it was successful. On day nine, we would come back for an ultrasound and blood work. We had mentioned several times before, but maybe this upcoming Christmas would be the last one with just the two of us. Maybe this was finally the beginning!

I didn't know what to expect when they finally grabbed us and brought us back into the surgical room for the transfer. The same bright lights were on, and the same calming music played in the background. Unfamiliar faces in the sea of support people moved around. Luckily our primary IVF doctor was there.

As they guided me into the stirrups and positioned my butt where they wanted it, I couldn't help but feel excited, despite the diazepam they had me take beforehand.

Things seemed to go smoothly until the doctor seemed to run straight into my cervix. I flinched.

"Sorry," she mumbled and tried navigating the catheter via ultrasound.

Bang, bang, bang.

Again and again, she rammed into something in there that was not an entirely pleasant demarcation. The diazepam was definitely wearing off. The wonderful ultrasound tech reminded me to tap my toes when it got uncomfortable, so those puppies were moving so fast they'd make a drummer jealous. Josh was patting my hand soothingly and then would lean over to kiss my forehead in support when a soft expletive would slip out of the doctor's mouth.

She was having a hard time getting through my cervix.

I felt their request to have a full bladder might have unintended consequences for all of us. They said it would help position the uterus better for the transfer. I thought they were wrong.

I was told it was comparable to a pap smear. Nope. My legs were shaking from stress and discomfort.

I kept mentally repeating that it would be nothing compared to childbirth. That had become my mental catchphrase whenever something infertility-related would start to hurt. Just because that was true didn't make those moments any less painful, but I was trying to remind myself of the tentative light at the end of the tunnel... and was hoping it wasn't a train.

Once they got the catheter in, we watched them shoot the embryo into my uterus on the ultrasound screen. It was super cool watching it propel out of the catheter and into my uterus.

And just like that, boom! I was pregnant.

The infertility boards call it PUPO: Pregnant Until Proven Otherwise.

And for the first time in my life, I was pregnant!

I wanted to cry.

But I held it together and just stared at the screen.

The doctor handed me a 4x6 photo of the embryo from that morning and explained the location of the placenta cells vs. the baby cells. She outlined where they punctured initially for the biopsy and explained the logistics of the blastocyst structure.

We were in awe of our little embryo.

Hopefully, this was a 'sticky' embryo—meaning in the TTC world that it would 'stick' to my uterine lining and stick around and become a baby.

"You might have some bleeding later, but everything went fine, so we're going to roll you back to your room for a twenty-minute rest, and I want you to stay laying on your back and take it easy for a bit."

The entire internet was full of people constantly arguing about whether laying prone was a factor in successful implantation. I'm not sure there was conclusive evidence one way or another, but it certainly couldn't hurt. Plus, I had no problem basking in my pregnancy for twenty minutes.

Then the most extended wait of my life began.

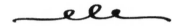

I spent the next week trying to take it as easy as possible to give the embryo its best chance at embedding itself in my uterine wall to set up camp. I had a bit of bleeding after the transfer for a day or two, but was used to randomly spotting, so I wasn't overly concerned. Plus, I remembered the doctor's warning that there might be spotting due to their troubles getting up into my uterus, so I chose not to panic.

The wait was brutal. I tried everything I could think of to keep my mind from obsessing. There were boards and boards online with ideas on how to pass the infamous TWW. Truthfully, not much helped.

I put the photograph of our embryo in a pretty silver photo frame and put it on the bookshelf I painted in our soon-to-be nursery. We had bought the crib when we first started TTC but hadn't assembled it. As years passed us by, it became more and more depressing to be in that room. We also purchased a rocking recliner at the same time. It was in the corner of the room, ready for a baby to soothe. Now that we had hit the pinnacle of infertility treatments though, we were going to have a baby soon, so Josh and I assembled the crib. We hung the artwork with lyrics to "A thousand years" by Christina Perri. I bought adorable sports-themed photos and put them in beautiful wood-accented frames. The white crib, grey walls, neutral carpet, and natural wood accents made the nursery tie together in such a pretty way. At night, after work, I'd go in there and sit on the chair, rocking while I looked at the room, imagining the day when my arms weren't empty.

I was ready.

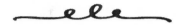

I wasn't ready.

I had been peeing on pregnancy test after pregnancy test at home for the last week and didn't have the slightest hint of a second line.

I know they said not to test at home, but from everything I was reading online, it looked like some women may test positive at home after Day Six or Seven so obviously I wanted to try too.

And I tried everything.

I used flashlights, the bright windows, holding it up under the bathroom lights, and more and still couldn't see even a faint second line. In the infertility world, there was such a prevalence of this that there were acronyms for this behavior. VVFL was for a very, very faint line. VVVFL was for a very, very, very faint line. And VVVVFL was for... you guessed it: very, very, very, very faint line. There was an entire corner of the internet devoted to hopeful moms looking for others to look at pictures of their pregnancy tests and tell them that others saw what they could not. There was also another very common phrase: Line Eyes. Line eyes are what you develop when you hope beyond hope that you're seeing a second line, but in reality, it's a lot of hope and imagination, but not reality.

There's also a corner of the infertility world that has helpful souls willing to take your photo of your pregnancy test and invert the colors. The theory behind that is that the inverted colors will help reveal a second line that your eyes might not see.

Not sure about the truth of that, but regardless, I was doing all of that anyway.

The rest of the hopeful moms agreed: no second line for me.

The interesting and frustrating thing about the Two Week Wait is that you begin developing all the symptoms of being pregnant due to all the hormones. So when I developed sore boobs and started getting tired on Day Six post-transfer, I wanted to shout from the rooftops. But even with all that, I just didn't feel pregnant.

We drove down after our two-week wait (TWW) was up and went in for my bloodwork. The drive down was somber. We did the same song and dance that we had done countless times before, and waited for them to call my name. I gave my blood to one of my favorite phlebotomists, who always used small needles on me.

Even though we weren't overly hopeful, we still grabbed a date at IHOP before we headed home. We enjoyed each other's company over some delicious pancakes and just tried to accept the results that we felt were coming.

Sure enough, that afternoon, we received the results that our baby boy did not stick.

Even though I thought I had prepared myself for that phone call over the last few days by looking at those negative tests and repeating it to myself over and over... the call still wrecked me.

I guess I still had a kernel of hope.

Shame on me.

Twenty-Three

THE IVF DOCTOR CALLED me a couple of days after our August 25 bloodwork results and discussed next steps. We agreed on doing another cycle after this next period was over and aiming for a September transfer.

The doc suggested we switch over to intramuscular progesterone rather than the suppositories, and I was good with that. The suppositories were messy and disgusting. Not to mention that the mess in my underwear made me think I wasn't absorbing as much of the drug as I needed to be. Who knew if that was accurate or not, but that's where my mind went when I saw all that mush from the progesterone suppository in my underwear. TMI, I know.

To put it in perspective, when I first saw the progesterone needles in the mail, I immediately texted Josh the following words: "I changed my mind. I don't want kids that bad. Fuck this."

I was obviously joking... but the fear of those needles was very real.

And apparently well deserved.

The progesterone shots were the worst shots I ever had. The oil was thick, and they required thicker needles. Also, we learned this the hard way–if you didn't massage the area after injecting the shot, you'd develop a lump of progesterone under the skin that would be sore to touch. Another bonus (read the sarcasm there) was that the oil would occasionally seep back out of the needle site. Because the oil was so thick, Josh would have to force the plunger down to get the oil to inject into the upper part of my butt. It was terrible. It was also different from the other shots because rather than pinching the site, you had to stretch the skin while injecting. Oh my god, it hurt so badly while being injected. God help me if Josh injected the progesterone shot in a lump from a previous night that we didn't break up. I would sob in pain. There were many nights that I sat on a lacrosse ball trying to massage the oil in and then promptly moved over to sit on a heating pad.

We learned if we wrapped the progesterone needle in the heating pad before injecting, the oil seemed to go in easier. But that was after a lot of trial and error. (Side note for the reader–I'm years out from these progesterone shots, IVF in my rearview mirror, and I STILL have some leftover progesterone lumps in my upper buttocks, so that's fun...).

What was even more frustrating than having to do shots every night again was the fact that every single time I spoke to any of the nurses at the clinic (whether in person or via phone), they always forgot that they had switched me over to the progesterone in oil (PIO) rather than the suppositories. Every single time. I constantly had to correct them. It was frustrating and made me feel like they didn't even bother to look at my chart before calling me. One nurse even suggested switching me over to PIO and I had to interrupt her and say that I was already doing that.

It doesn't give you warm fuzzies when your trusted medical team keeps messing that up.

I called them a week before my transfer saying that I was experiencing some brown spotting but was told not to worry–the hormones could do that. When it switched to bright red blood, I got concerned. I called again, and they said not to worry. The concern intensified when the bright red blood continued for the third day. I don't think they were worried at all, but let me come in anyway so they could look. They performed an ultrasound and some bloodwork to ensure everything was all right. There was nothing remarkable that would indicate why I was bleeding. The ultrasound tech mentioned that my lining looked okay and that I had a "triple-A lining," whatever that meant. She saw some cervical polyps, and her best guess was that those were causing the bleeding. She didn't seem overly concerned. They put me on antibiotics just in case anything was brewing and to help if I had any type of inflammation in my uterus.

They said that I could go to the clinic in Greenfield on Tuesday for bloodwork and that I didn't have to go all the way back to Springfield. So that was a small win.

This transfer was like my first. I received a nice pill to take about thirty minutes before our arrival time which was supposed to calm my nerves. I brought a big water bottle so my bladder could be nice and full to allow a more manageable insertion. Josh donned his scrubs while I gowned up, and we anxiously waited for them to get to us. For this morning, we were in Recovery Room Two, which I thought was a good sign. A new room, new experience, so hopefully... a new result.

As they wheeled me in, I remembered the discomfort from my previous experience, and you could hear my heart rate spike a little on the monitor. The same bright lights, similar soft music, and the same cold stirrups awaited me. This time I brought cute custom socks with me that said, "It's my Transfer day!" So those were keeping my piggies warm during the procedure.

They plopped the little embryo in with little fanfare, and wheeled me back out to relax and let the little embryo stick to whatever uterine lining he could find.

I brought my now-empty photo frame for the new embryo picture of our potential future little baby.

As we once again left the clinic, I stared at the embryo picture in my hand, excited about what the future might hold and looking forward to peeing on a stick in a couple of days.

Waiting and patience were never my strengths, and I never said they were.

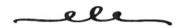

When I started having spotting three days after my transfer, I worried. When the spotting turned into heavy brown bleeding a couple of days later, I resigned myself to another loss.

I did my due diligence: I peed on my sticks.

But I wasn't inverting any photos in photo apps.

I wasn't asking the infertility warriors online for their opinions on whether they saw a second line.

I just knew it.

My lining wasn't ready. I should have listened to my gut.

And because I didn't, I lost our baby girl.

Our one chance of having a baby girl was gone because I didn't advocate for myself and push back on them when I felt the bleeding was too heavy

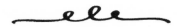

On September 29, we received the results that both of us were expecting, given I was still bleeding and it had become a period.

Not pregnant

I couldn't even cry.

We did something different with this transfer by not telling anyone that we were doing it. It was stressful during the first transfer when my mom, who had a heart of gold and just wanted to know, would ask what was happening. She was calling me almost every day for medical updates. It was frustrating because, as an IVF patient, there wasn't a bunch that I was told, so there wasn't much to relay. It was a lot of 'hurry to wait.' People who golf would thrive in IVF.

My poor mother. My absolute hero. The person who was an absolute rock and unwaveringly supportive was enduring my frustrations and fear. It was like she triggered something in me. If she called after an appointment, I instantly would become defensive and snap at her. She was always asking legitimate questions—I had usually asked myself—but somehow, her asking those questions would trigger a reaction in me that was bitchy and ungrateful. I would snap an "I don't know!"

I didn't know.

Her asking just seemed to remind me how much I didn't know and how alone I was in all of this. And when it was right after an appointment, like Josh and I were still in the car, and I'd get a call, I'd just snap and go mental on her like an unstable psychopath. Basically, biting the most reliable and caring hand in the world to have ever fed me. It made little sense! And I knew I was being irrational and that I was being oversensitive: That I was being a jerk. But it was building up in me. All this anger and frustration. And exhaustion. I lashed out. And bless my mother. The woman was a saint. Because she continued to reach out, she continued to support me. She continued to try to understand what I was going through. Even though I was a total wretch and a goblin every time, she tried. And even after I'd try to tell myself not to snap the next time she asked something, I would. And I'd feel terrible and frustrated, but she'd never make me feel bad. She was unwavering and incredible. And the unsung hero of my life story.

Therefore, we did things differently this second transfer. We told no one, *except maybe two friends.*

Besides that, no one knew we were doing this transfer, so we wouldn't be asked questions that stressed us (read: me) out.

The doctor wondered if maybe I had chronic endometritis. From what I gathered, this was an inflammation of the uterine lining. She ordered an endometrial biopsy to get a sample of the uterus lining to check. If I had that, I would need to be given antibiotics (Doxycycline) to clear it up before my next transfer. I clarified that they had already put me on antibiotics for the second transfer, so shouldn't that have taken care of any possible endometritis? She seemed surprised on the phone. Again, I felt like I constantly had to remind them what they had prescribed me. She brushed off the reminder that I had already tried antibiotics with a "we can try that again, and this time we can also try some steroids. It's been shown to help sometimes to suppress inflammation."

Ultimately, she said that she thinks it's a lining issue. A part of me was doing an 'I told you so' dance in my head. I always knew something weird was going on in my uterus: with all my heavy periods and the fact that they were so irregular and inconsistent. Maybe *this* was our golden ticket?

But by this point, I was also worrying about non-infertility-related things.

The CPA firm that purchased my old firm had approached me about returning. I missed my client mix and the work I was doing. I also missed the work-life balance I had. This last tax season had been so exhausting. Ranging anywhere between sixty to eighty-hour weeks, I was still burnt out, and it was almost October. I didn't necessarily want to leave. I had a good gig going, and I liked my boss and some of my co-workers. But the switch to hourly left a sour taste in my mouth, and I felt unappreciated. Now, after two failed cycles, I was trying to look ahead and plan.

Famous last words, I know.

It seemed like whenever I tried to have a plan, life threw me a curve ball and laughed at me.

But damn it, I was going to try!

Perseverance!

So even though I was benefiting from infertility benefits (to an extent), I was also draining whatever PTO and savings we had to do these infertility treatments. If we did another cycle, I'd be out of my PTO time and not have anything left for maternity leave.

It was almost kind of funny. I used to want to plan my pregnancies around tax season because I didn't want to do that to any employer of mine. Abandon them during the busiest part of the year. But now?

Now, I didn't care. I didn't care when I got pregnant or when I was due. I just wanted a baby. If my employer wasn't cool with the due date? Then, okay. So be it.

I was internally warring with myself about the pros and cons of switching jobs. I agreed to come in for a quick interview and meet and greet. It went great. After saying goodbye and thank you to the staff who took me out to lunch, they handed me a packet with an offer letter inside. I was elated!

That is until I saw that the offer was even less than I was making now.

After discussing with Josh, I asked for a higher salary range because if I was going to be losing infertility benefits and taking a pay cut... that made my decision super easy. No contest. Thanks for the offer, but I'm not looking to leave a job I'm fine with to make less money and worse benefits.

Ultimately, after a couple of back and forths, we just couldn't agree on a salary. So I said I wasn't ready to make a move, and thanked them for their time and for thinking of me.

Josh and I went ahead with our IVF plans. In the third week of my cycle, on October 9, we went in for my endometrial biopsy. It was one of the more painful procedures I had done. We drove down to Burr Medical, and I loaded myself into the stirrups. Then I experienced enough pain during the biopsy that I was moaning and whimpering as I pushed myself up onto the bed, trying to get away.

When they were done and I was left sobbing on the table, Josh grabbed some tissues and wiped my sweaty brow and tear-stained cheeks. I had to take a few minutes to get myself under control, and once I did, realized what that must have sounded like to the poor parents to be that were walking past our door.

The thought quickly faded once Josh helped me off the table, and I looked back and saw the blood-soaked paper covering it. I wanted to vomit... and cry. I was just so tired of all of this.

I was sick and tired of being sick and tired.

But then, if this is what it took to be a mom...

"It's worth every heartache," I reminded myself weakly.

Twenty-Four

As luck would have it, the CPA firm reached back within a week with a new offer. One that made it a much harder decision. As Josh and I made my standard pro versus con list, I realized how nice it would be to have 100% paid medical time. If we continued with IVF, which was honestly up in the air, then paid time off would be incredible. I was feeling burnt out and exhausted from the treatments. So, I wasn't sure if I wanted to take a break from all the procedures for a while or not. My emotions and hormones weren't my own anymore. Sore boobs, random bleeding, hot flashes galore. You name it; I had it. Plus, I was just exhausted. I had developed dark(er) circles under my eyes and had trouble sleeping. Depression reared its head and set its sights on me.

Once we had the new offer in hand and the pro/con list finished, it seemed like the obvious choice. Giving my notice was one of the harder and more unpleasant things I had to do so far in my life. However, infertility had a way of putting things into perspective. I muscled through that unpleasant experience and rallied my unpredictable emotions.

The meeting didn't go well. My boss didn't handle it well, and I responded in kind. We both handled it poorly, and I awkwardly left the office and headed back to my own.

My original plan was to provide them with a three weeks' notice, which I did. But after a day or two of awkwardly working and avoiding my boss, I was asked to leave without completing the remaining time. There's a big fear in public accounting that you'll take information or clients with you. I didn't have any desire to do that, but when anyone goes to a competitor, no matter the industry, I think that's just standard practice. Knowing this, I packed up my stuff and headed home.

Now that I had some free time on my hands, Josh and I discussed our next steps in Mission: Become Parents. I reached out to the IVF clinic and asked for the latest test results. The results from the endometrial biopsy had come back clear. It wasn't endometritis.

"Okay, so it's not endometritis... then why can't I get pregnant with perfectly healthy embryos?" By now, I was feeling very good about our decision to go with the PGS testing, so they couldn't blame this on unhealthy embryos incorrectly.

"Well, our technician mentioned that she might have seen a polyp on your cervix during one of the ultrasounds, which could prevent implantation. With this sort of thing, we never know for sure what's going on, but we do our best guess and go from there."

But did she really? Or are you guys also grasping at straws?

"Okay, so on that note, I'm going to be changing jobs and losing the little coverage we have for infertility treatments. So, Josh and I talked, and we want to do another retrieval before it is switched. We've always wanted more than two kids, so we'll have to do it again anyway, and it would be better to do it now when we don't have to juggle other children and while we still have insurance." Inwardly, the superstitious part of me (that was never really that big) was wondering if my first round of eggs was a bad batch and if none of them would stick. Also, I didn't want to have to deal with Retrievals and all the monitoring that went along with it when Josh and I had a toddler running around at home. A small part of me was hoping we'd get another shot at a girl. The way I phrased it to her was more like telling and less like asking. I was learning to be my own advocate, damn it.

"Sure, we can do that. Let us know when."

I blinked. I didn't think it would actually work.

"Though I believe we should schedule surgery to inspect that polyp that we noticed on your cervix. There's no way of knowing if that is affecting your implantation results, but it's something we can try to remove and see what happens. Again, there's no guarantee, but just something else we can try."

I could hear the tentative hope in her voice that maybe this was the winning ticket for us. Even though I was tired and just wanted a baby, this was just another step towards getting one. So if that's what I needed to do, then I would do it.

"Okay, let's get that scheduled."

"Let me get a nurse on the line to schedule things with you." As they put me on hold, I hummed quietly along with the music I had become all too familiar with. I think at that point, I had heard that music more than my actual radio stations.

"Hi, Ashley? Dr. Sadia tells me you want to schedule a polyp removal surgery?"

"Yes, but I need to schedule another retrieval first."

"Oh! I thought you still had some embryos remaining... let me see..." I interrupted her as I heard her rapidly flipping through the chart.

"I have embryos remaining, but like I told Dr. Sadia, I'm losing my infertility benefits and changing jobs, and we want more than two kids anyway, so it's easier to do a retrieval now rather than three years from now."

"Okay, sure, sure. Some insurances require you to use up any remaining embryos before letting you do another retrieval, so you'll want to double-check your particular policy before—"

"Yeah, I called them this morning and asked. They're looking into it, but the agent on the phone thinks it's okay to do another retrieval. She's going to confirm. However, she mentioned that I only qualify for partial coverage on six IVF cycles. She didn't seem to know what that meant. Like... was the retrieval itself a complete cycle, even though there wasn't a transfer? Or does each frozen transfer count as an IVF cycle? Or does it only cover me for six retrievals?" I was hoping the nurse could shed some light on what a "complete cycle" meant.

"I actually do not know what they consider a complete cycle. We rarely deal with the insurance piece. We only usually call them to appeal to different things similar to what we did for you regarding the estrogen limits and other prescription-related items. If you hold on a minute, I'll track down Dr. Sadia again and ask her quickly to see if she knows."

As I waited, I bobbed my knee while staring at the girls on the hockey field running laps. I was coaching again and managing work. Everything was exhausting, especially today, where I tried my best to coordinate visits, insurance, treatment, and life. Coaching was fulfilling but also stressful at times. Not just for the coaching aspect, but for trying to manage my cycle and symptoms simultaneously. Things like: having to play phone tag when I had a big bleed that day or if we had a game far away that would bring us home at the upper limit of my shot window.

Worth every headache, I reminded myself.

"Okay," she started in my ear. "Dr. Sadia said she doesn't know what insurance considers a full cycle, and you should call our insurance coordinator to check with her."

"Oh... all righty. I'll call her next, then..." Guess the girls were going to be assigned a couple more laps.

"But let's get that retrieval and polyp removal scheduled in the meantime. When were you thinking?"

I outlined my desire to do another retrieval for the beginning of December, assuming my period cooperated and came as scheduled. There was never much predictability to it in the timing or the duration. Sometimes I spotted for days before actually starting. This caused the beginning sensation of a slight headache as the nurse reminded me to call on Day One.

What did they consider Day One?

"Also, rather than fighting with insurance non-stop for this cycle, is there a way that we can just get estrogen pills rather than patches? It was a nightmare to manage to schedule and pay for the boxes last time."

"Sure, we can put in an order for the estrogen pills. We rarely prescribe those as people seem to get more side effects with those–headaches and weight gain being the main ones reported, but I can put an order in for those if you'd like."

I breathed a sigh of relief. Those pills would last me longer and be a zillion times cheaper than the patches. Not to mention the lower stress level that would come with them. Worth whatever weight gain and headaches were coming my way.

We then scheduled the polyp removal for a couple of weeks later, on December 21. The timing would work out because Josh and I would be home for Christmas the next couple of days after, so if recovery was unpleasant, I wouldn't miss any time at my new job–which I was to start on December 11.

The 'turn this frown upside down' part of me was relieved that I could do the retrieval in between my job switch. Given how rough it was the first time, I expected a week or so of recovery. Now that they knew how my body responded to the hormones, they could tweak the dosages and whatnot to cater to my response. I was hoping for a few healthy embryos we could put in storage and use later. When I told my new boss I had the surgery coming up, she suggested pushing my start date back to account for the recovery time and I appreciated that. I thought it would work in our favor.

On day one of my cycles, I received my marching orders to call and that I'd be on the Birth Control Lupron Protocol again. They'd send me my handwritten calendar in the mail with my important dates and monitoring visits shortly. Then we were off. The next phase begins in three... two... one.

Calling the insurance coordinator was frustrating. She told me I needed to call insurance to ask what a complete cycle was considered. Was it: a retrieval and a fresh transfer? Was it: just a retrieval? Was it: just a frozen transfer? I told her I already had and that they told me to talk to her. Luckily, she said she'd try to call and get a more concrete answer, but I wasn't so sure.

She said she saw different treatments on what a complete cycle was. Some insurance companies viewed FETs (frozen embryo transfers) as complete cycles, but others didn't include FETs at all, and you could do those all day long until the cows came home. Regardless, she said she'd call and ask. She also dropped a bomb on me that my cross-border referral was expiring on November 24, so I needed to call my PCP to ask for that to be renewed. In the meantime, she'd request a pre-authorization from insurance for another retrieval.

Another lap girls while Coach tries to place another IVF-related phone call.

It was okay. They needed the conditioning.

As I played phone tag with my PCP office for the rest of practice, I finally received lackluster news. Apparently, they couldn't extend my cross-border referral until the previous one expired. So I had to wait until November 24 and then call on November 27 when they opened back up and requested a new one. This would drive my insurance company nuts, and we'd have to resubmit everything, especially with me being mid-cycle.

But c'est la vie.

Josh and I were discussing the option of transferring both final embryos at the same time. Online, I saw better odds of getting pregnant if we transferred both. And if we were down to the wire with our remaining cycles, then transferring both would get us the most bang for our buck. I didn't particularly rejoice at the idea of being pregnant with twins. But having a baby or babies was what this was all about, and if the choice was having no kids versus having twins, well, we know the decision was a no-brainer.

Twins all day.

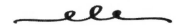

A couple of weeks later, on October 30, I received my letter in the mail from my insurance.

They had approved the request for another retrieval cycle.

Cue the waterworks and waves of relief.

And so began another series of stimulation hormones.

A little before five in the morning on December 3, we woke up bright and early to head in for our retrieval.

After we got down there and set up in Room One, I changed into the hospital johnny and got comfortable. I tried to embrace the valium they gave me so I could remain calm for this surgery. Josh had forgotten not to put on deodorant that morning, so I spent ten minutes teasing him about his carcinogenic armpits and what that would do to my egg quality. As we were chuckling, Dr. Sadia poked her head in.

"Oh, it's you guys! I'll be in charge of the surgeries today!"

We blinked in surprise. We knew that already. She told us each time we saw her that week.

"Uh... yeah, I think you mentioned that," Josh added.

"Oh, great! And we're doing a fresh transfer today, correct?"

My stomach dropped. "No! No, we're not. We're doing the retrieval, and then they're being frozen, so we can do the hysteroscopy for the polyp search in a couple of weeks, right?" The heart rate monitor started beeping a little faster.

"Oh, yes! You're right! You're freezing this batch. And doing PGS testing again?"

Another strike.

"No... No, we're not doing testing this round, either." I had many occasions to be less than impressed with the bedside manner of my doctor, and this was just another shining example of how she didn't know who I was. They better be using Josh's semen to fertilize the correct embryos in a couple of hours...

"Oh, right! Of course, I forgot about that. Yes, I think we'll start seeing better results once we get the polyp removed. Okay, I'm heading back. A nurse will be in a minute to prep you. Has the Anesthesiologist come in to see you yet?"

I desperately hoped it wasn't the same person from the last retrieval. That one was a pompous prick. And I didn't think that lightly. We could overhear him at the nurses' station rambling on about a fancy dinner party he went to the night before and how there was another person there that was so "garrulous and loquacious." Then he paused dramatically and asked the surrounding nurses, "do you know what that means?" then condescendingly gave them Webster's definitions. Josh and I had looked at each other in disgust when we overheard this. What a douche canoe!

I was hoping this was a different one.

Thankfully it was.

A few minutes after my super nice nurse gave me a hand IVF, the anesthesiologist came in and started running through the questions. It was seven-thirty, so it was early, but the man was a grouch. I tried to crack some jokes and talk about my nerves concerning the surgery and recovery, and he didn't even respond to my comments. He just stared at his clipboard and only asked the questions on the board, and if I mentioned anything else, he pretended I had said nothing. I looked at Josh and ground my teeth. He smiled placatingly and patted my hand.

My nurse wheeled me back into the surgery room and tried to distract me as she heard my heart rate increase once again. She had given me some lidocaine in my hand when I told her my hand ached the entire time during our last retrieval, so I thought that was a nice touch. Now that we were back in the operating room, she also put an oxygen mask on me as they got me into position. She patted my hand and talked about Christmas shopping and how she had a claustrophobia attack while at the mall the night before. Her rambling didn't quite take away the nerves, but I appreciated it. Plus, I enjoyed thinking about something else.

As they injected my elbow with the same meds as last time, I didn't experience the same level of fire. The first time I questioned ever doing IVF, this round wasn't actually all that terrible. I do not know if they did a different speed, a different dose, or if it was the oxygen, but whatever it was, it helped.

Within minutes swift blackness claimed me.

I came to consciousness mid-sentence. Talking about God knows what.

Josh was sitting next to my head, playing with my hair, and they reclined me with loads of warmed blankets. Dr. Sadia popped her head in and said everything went well. I had twelve follicles and twelve eggs. She said that they'd see how many were mature in a couple of hours, and in four hours, they'd use ICSI to fertilize them.

That made my sluggish brain pause.

Earlier that week, when the ultrasound tech was reading our numbers, I remember having embryos on one side but not that many on the left side. The sizes that she gave us weren't super awesome. I knew for the first round, most of the eggs were in the high teens when we triggered. Or at least, I thought they were. But this time, it seemed like I had eggs of all different sizes. The tech had measured the ones on my right side, ranging from 9mm to 14mm to 17mm. Josh and I had gone home and hoped we wouldn't get instructions to trigger because the follicles still seemed too small. But when we received our instructions, we assumed that the bloodwork must have shown something to reflect that we should be triggering. But now? Now that she implied the eggs weren't mature... Maybe we misheard her...

Or maybe we triggered too early...

"Hey hon, how are you feeling?" Super Nice Nurse came back in to check on me.

"Pretty good! Slight cramping on the right side, but I'm feeling pretty awesome, actually. Thanks again for not making the hand IVF hurt." I have a thing with needles and veins. It stresses me out. So having her take that care and make it not unpleasant for every waking second was truly appreciated.

"No problem, hon. Alright, well, you look great, so you're free to go whenever! Here's your discharge paperwork."

As she started reading the discharge instructions to Josh and me, we were chatting about grabbing breakfast and relaxing today. We talked about OHSS, our night plans, and what to look out for. But then my right side started screaming.

"Woah hon, you all right?"

I grabbed the bar next to me and bit my lip. My forehead broke out into a cold sweat, and a soft moan came from me.

Josh stood up next to me and glanced over at the nurse. "What's happening?"

"Hold on a second," she said, looking up at my vitals on the cart next to me. "Her face lost all color, and her lips started turning white. I'm grabbing the doc." She left.

The pain was intense. It was all focused on my right side, which felt like my right ovary. Did it rupture? Could that even happen? My body shook with the pain, and Josh wiped the sweat dripping from my face as my body seized and caught fire.

The nurse came back in and brought a heating pad and more warmed blankets. She piled them on me and murmured softly about the anesthesiologist already being in the OR with the next patient, so she couldn't get a prescription for any pain meds. She said that we'd have to wait it out until he was out.

In truth, I wasn't processing her words. All my focus was internally on the stabbing pain in my side. My eyes rolled back in my head, and I briefly lost consciousness. Josh grabbed my shoulder to bring me back. It happened a couple more times before I was hit with a wave of nausea that had me clenching my teeth, so I didn't vomit everywhere. This couldn't be normal. Did the surgery go bad? Did something go wrong?!

The nurse came back after a few minutes which felt like hours with a prescription for Percocet and some antinausea meds. The anesthesiologist had mentioned something about me already receiving fentanyl during the surgery, so they had to be aware of what they were prescribing me for the pain and nausea. Again, I wasn't really coherent. I didn't care. I just wanted to hear that this happened sometimes and that I wasn't dying in my pursuit of being a mom.

And apparently, I wasn't dying because, after ten minutes, she came back in and remarked reassuringly, "You look much better. You have your color back."

The meds helped. The fire had subsided to low cramping, and the nausea went away. As the nurse was chit-chatting with us to get a pulse for how I was feeling, Dr. Sadia, popped her head in and said, "oh, you're still here?"

Josh glared at her from his place at my sweat-soaked head.

After what I just went through, combined with all the hormones rushing through my system. I didn't need to hear that. But it only got worse.

We heard another patient check in at the desk across from our Room One curtain and listened to the nurse there tell them that there would be a room available soon, but they'd have to wait out in reception.

Well, that was a trigger for good ol' Grouchy Anesthesiologist. Because then, he popped his head into our room, looked at me reclining in the bed under a pile of blankets, and said drily, "oh, Number One is still here," and then walked back out into the hall, saying loudly, "this is going to push us back, guys."

My blood boiled.

Anger, stress, and pain all made me cry.

I'm a crier.

But I'm also known for having an occasional bitch-bone. I usually keep that reserved for my inner monologue and Josh, but I felt attacked.

Scratch that.

I was in pain. I felt frustrated. I felt scared. I felt exhausted. I felt unimportant. Most importantly, I felt attacked.

I was gearing up to rage.

I pushed up in bed with a fire in my heart, ready to go to bat for all the future women that had to cycle through this anesthesiologist and how insensitive that comment was.

We were here because of infertility! It's not like we wanted to be here! And it's not like I was here in this room for the room service! I just had a terrible last twenty minutes. And for him to say something like that?!

My future Mama Bear was ready to rock.

Josh stopped it.

He pushed my shoulder back against the bed and tried quickly to calm me down. The super nice nurse came in as he was trying to diffuse the emotional bomb that I had become and quickly joined in.

"Ignore him, hon. He's a jerk."

I quelled my raging fire, but as we left the building and I waddled into the parking lot, I started crying.

I was on a pendulum every single day, every single minute. This was just too much in one direction.

Why did people have to be so insensitive?

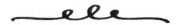

"Hi Ashley, how are you feeling today?" My favorite nurse chirped in my ear the next morning.

"Oh my God. It's like night and day. I feel so much better this time than I did last time! It's crazy!"

"It's so strange how that happens. We always wonder if it's the location of the follicles, the anesthesia, or a number of other things. But I'm glad you're feeling better!" I hummed in agreement. I was feeling fantastic compared to the last time. "So you had twelve eggs retrieved. Only nine were mature, and only five fertilized." I swallowed the lump in my throat, giving watery eyes to Josh. "The lab is going to monitor them and watch as they grow and develop and will call you on Day Three, which will be Wednesday. They'll let you know on Friday and Saturday what has been frozen. And if you wanted to do genetic screening again, they would do that on Friday and Saturday."

"Okay, yeah, if there is still the 40% attrition rate of those remaining five, then it will be only one or two embryos, and it makes little sense to pay for the biopsying and testing of just one or two, so I'll let you know." I've given up trying to remind them about things I've said and the medications I was on. Josh and I were looking at other infertility clinics in the two-hour radius around our home that we could switch to if this was yet another failed cycle. Someplace that made me feel a little less like a number and more like a person.

As luck would have it, Day Three was pretty good news. Four embryos were still alive and kicking. We didn't have a big drop-off, and I felt cautiously optimistic about it all. That dropped a little on Day Five when they told us that only three embryos were still developing. But Josh kept me positive by calling them the Big Three.

Then, on Day Six, we got the call that only *one* was left and able to be frozen.

One.

A small part of my heart died right then and there.

"It's better than none." Josh weakly tried to encourage me. But even he was feeling the pressure of all of this.

To be honest, I was tired.

... burnt out.

Not just regular-tired. Bone-deep-tired.

The hormones were hitting me, and I just wanted to curl up into a ball and sleep. Sleep for a week. A month. A year. I didn't want to do anything. I didn't want to have to do anything. I was feeling tired, but I was also feeling angry. How can all these people have these easy times getting pregnant, and here I was, having to do IVF? At this point, I wasn't even trying to fight off the judgmental thoughts. How could people just get knocked up so easily? What were they drinking, and where could I get some? Was it in the water? Was one of my Facebook friends correct that we did this to ourselves by using scented soap and deodorant with aluminum? Was another one of my so-called friends correct, and maybe there was a reason that my egg and his sperm couldn't produce a baby? Was she right, and were we really messing with the normal scheme of things? I was just so tired. It shouldn't be this hard for me. It shouldn't be this hard for us. I had worked so hard in life to bring us to a point where we would be great parents and be able to provide a baby with an awesome life... and here we were. It wasn't supposed to be this hard.

And I was alone.

I knew a couple of people at this point who had done IVF. All four of them had ended up with a baby of their own. So they always offered hope. But I felt so stressed and pessimistic at this point. It was so discouraging to have a roadblock at every turn. I would just love one week of not having to advocate for myself or fight for something.

I kept trying to remind myself it was good parenting prep. The pain from the shots was good preparation for the pains of childbirth. It was good practice for being pregnant to experience headaches, nausea, and vomiting. The advocating piece was good practice for being a parent.

But again, I was tired and hormonal, and to make matters worse, I'd immediately receive a phone call from my mom before I made it in the door sometimes. Out of love, she drilled me about what happened at the appointment and what such-and-such means. That she read XYZ online and... She just had so many questions. Most of the time, I didn't have an answer for her and that feeling of being unprepared made me snappy and grouchy. The stress of it all was getting to me, and I was becoming a person I didn't really like all that much anymore.

And now I had to face telling her we only had one embryo from this cycle. I would have to deal with the resulting "whys" coming my way. I just wasn't in the headspace to answer her nicely because I didn't know why either.

The doctors had no discernable reason as to why IVF wasn't working, given that *I* had no diagnosed condition. Everyone said the problem was *Josh*. Based on what they said during appointments, this should have been a slam dunk. Yet, here we were.

What if IVF never worked for us? What if we never have kids?

So maybe I'd call my mom and give her an update after I took a restorative nap.

A long, depressing nap.

Twenty-Five

I STARTED MY NEW job on December 11. I was completely recovered from my retrieval and ready to rock. No OHSS. No residual pain and discomfort. An altogether different experience.

I had my hysteroscopy polypectomy scheduled and a tentative date for my final FET. Josh and I had officially decided that we'd try to transfer the newest embryo to mix up our juju, and if it didn't work, then we'd look into having a consultation with another IVF clinic.

We made this decision because there was no reason given to us as to why a perfectly healthy twenty-seven-year-old female couldn't get pregnant. We wanted a bit more than "idiopathic infertility." Even though that might be a legitimate diagnosis, I didn't feel well cared for. So we'd try somewhere else instead of wasting another embryo at this clinic.

The hysteroscopic polypectomy was one of the more benign surgeries I'd had. It was at a surgical center rather than through the IVF clinic, and I was put completely under during the procedure. Josh had to watch a surgery board to see where I was in the surgical process. Once he was paged and brought back into my recovery booth, it quickly moved. I came out of anesthesia like usual–chatty and disoriented but relatively chipper. Dr. Sadia came out with some pictures for us of my cervix and couldn't find a picture of the polyp she said they had removed. Who knows what happened in there, but besides being sore and groggy, I was ready to leave.

I remember little of the recovery process. It was one of the rather uneventful parts of our infertility journey. I was so used to things going haywire that it was a welcomed reprieve, actually.

Because the surgery was scheduled for week three of my cycle, I didn't have to wait long for the next phase to begin, which was our final FET before we threw in the towel and took some time off from the whole hormonal process.

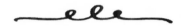

January 5 brought my period and the excitement (and slight dread), of knowing this was our last cycle before a break. At this point, it was all out of pocket, as I had changed insurance when I changed jobs. So maybe it was for the best that this would be the final go-round. Not only for the financial break but the hormonal and emotional break as well. I was trying to moderate my mood swings the last couple of weeks, and with tax season right around the corner at this new firm, I needed to be in tiptop shape.

With this FET cycle, I only had to worry about taking the estrogen pills for the first few weeks. So that was nice getting a break from the shots and giving my bruised and swollen belly and butt a chance to recover.

I developed some random spotting, which worried me based on how things went last time. But it wasn't nearly to the same degree as the bleeding before, so I made sure that I mentioned it to them frequently and had them be very thorough during our monitoring appointments. Also, the estrogen pills helped me pack on ten lbs. In just a couple of weeks, I was amazed. I didn't want or need that weight gain, but whatever it took—acne, headaches, hot flashes, cramping, spotting, and all.

Worth every shot. Worth every ache — both physical and of the heart. However, I did change many things during this cycle. I very much got in touch with my inner hippie during this last month. I bought essential oils that catered to infertility and the reproductive system. I diffused those and rubbed some on the heels of my feet before bed. I also practiced affirmations and positive thinking at least once a day that centered around being fertile. Josh and I also attended our first acupuncture session, during which he fell asleep, and I had a mini panic attack. I had to ring the bell to ask him to remove the needles because I was so overwhelmed. But I tried!

I was taking a daily aspirin as a blood thinner and drinking cranberry juice every day in an attempt to thicken my uterine lining.

I listened to positive pregnancy hypnosis podcasts and psyched myself up for this upcoming transfer.

I also had a couple of massages and had one scheduled for a couple of days after the transfer to help me relax further.

I was throwing all the spaghetti at the wall.

I even bought a pineapple so I could eat the core after the transfer to ingest some bromelain. I read online that it is an enzyme that could aid in implantation.

And, of course, I had my trusty rose quartz crystals from my friend right next to my head on my headboard every night. (I even 'charged' them up by leaving them under the light of a full moon... or something like that).

So even though there was not much science behind any of these individual theories–I figured, at this point, none of it could hurt. If my doctor wasn't demanding I stop any of it, I was doing it all.

Oh, and I also tried foot baths during the time in between my hysteroscopy and my period to try to suck out any impurities in my body. The bath water was truly disgusting. I'm not sure what was in there, I just know it was hideous, and if it truly was impurities and toxins in my body, then I didn't stand a chance during this cycle!

Regardless, I was still in a good headspace when we went to the transfer on January 26. I was wearing my 'Mother of Embryos' custom t-shirt, and I was repeating "third time's the charm" to every nurse I spoke to that day. I was all affirmations and positive vibes. I was projecting the crap out of it and into the universe.

Some examples of my affirmations:

It's going to work because:

I don't have a polyp on my cervix

    1. I experimented with yoga poses, continued going to the gym, and

had my friend come over and do some reiki on me.

2. A third IVF doctor I hadn't met yet did the transfer

3. I got to wear my shirt and bra the whole time

4. Josh got to wear pants under his scrubs

5. They let me play the lion king theme like when Rafiki brought in Simba

6. And that third IVF doctor that did the procedure had a cat named is Simba

7. The first transfer of 2018 for us

8. The realization that our sleep schedules are perfect for co-parenting

9. I never had jell-o after transfer before

10. Never took a three-hour nap after transfer before

11. TWW ends on Superbowl Sunday

12. Absolutely exhausted during the TWW

13. Pineapple after transfer to promote implantation

14. Chiropractor before transfer

15. Massage the week after transfer

16. Cranberry juice to thicken the lining

17. Essential oils

18. Baby aspirin

I had major cramping after the transfer, even though the doctor was super gentle with the speculum. At one point, she asked me if I wanted her to reduce the pressure a little, and then it felt much better. I felt like my comfort was a priority for her, and that it was. The two catheters going up felt like they ran into my uterine wall several times, and I would get some cramping. It felt like a bad period cramp after that. I took some extra strength Tylenol after.

The super nice nurse hugged me goodbye and wished us luck. "No insult, honey, but I hope I don't see you again!"

I spent the next nine days relaxing and throwing positive vibes into the universe.

I was absolutely 100% convinced that this would be *the* successful transfer. I started testing shortly after the transfer but wasn't receiving any positive home pregnancy tests. That was expected. However, I started spotting about two days after the transfer. They assured me again that it was from going up into the uterus and the irritation that the speculum and tubes caused, regardless I went for bloodwork. They wanted to test my progesterone and estrogen levels, but also threw in an early pregnancy test. No surprise, the hCG pregnancy blood test was negative, and luckily the rest of the bloodwork showed that nothing funky was going on.

Then, a couple of days later, I saw a very, very, very, faint line!

I was ecstatic! I couldn't believe my eyes. It was finally here!

I didn't tell Josh right away. I wanted to make sure that it got darker as the days progressed. Sure enough, the line did indeed get darker.

I finally spilled the beans one night before Josh was heading to soccer. Bad timing, I know. I spent the first year of our TTC journey looking at all the cute ways to announce. At the bottom of a coffee cup, a onesie left on the bed, a positive pregnancy test in a present box, etc. After a couple of years, I just didn't have it in me to prep something like that.

I confessed I had been getting faint positive on the HPT's and they had been progressively getting darker.

Josh thought I was joking at first. I wish I had recorded it - his reaction was precious. He just couldn't believe that I was pregnant. Frankly, neither could I.

As we jumped up and down in our kitchen, holding hands like madmen, I wondered if maybe there was something to the whole 'positive thinking' business. I found that my mood drastically improved, and I had more optimism in my heart again.

Maybe it was the polyp?

Or maybe it was our one and only lucky embryo from that second retrieval. Since we didn't do PGS testing, a part of me was convinced it was a girl, and the universe would laugh at us and give us a girl when we had resigned ourselves to boys. Either way, I was over the moon.

When we went in for our bloodwork on Super Bowl Sunday, February 4, Josh and I were relaxed and in good spirits. We knew we had this. We knew that it finally worked. My home pregnancy tests were very positive at this point. And I had bought several different brands to confirm. I tried digital. I tried pink dye. I tried blue dye. I tried rapid response. I tried early detection. I tried them all. And every single one came back positive.

When the time came for us to do our bloodwork at Burr Medical, Josh and I knew that I was pregnant and had no nerves at all. I chatted animatedly with the phlebotomists and smiled at everyone in sight. I wasn't just PUPO. I was proven! Plus, I had sore boobs and cramping, and slight spotting. If it quacks like a duck and walks like a duck.... Ya know?

We did our bloodwork and left the hospital.

Josh looked over at me and happily asked, "Pancakes?"

We went to IHOP for some delicious pancakes and conversation while we waited for the inevitable phone call that we were finally pregnant. Then we'd tell our families.

We got home late that morning and decided to take a little siesta while we waited for the doctor to call. The Patriots weren't playing until six thirty, so we had loads of time to kill. I thought gleefully, who knows when the next time we could nap like this once the baby was here?

When I received a phone call in the middle of our nap, I shot up in bed. Josh pulled out his phone, put it on record, and pointed it at me so we could document this monumental occasion.

"Hello?"

"Um, yes, is this Ashley?" I heard in my ear.

"Yup!" I said giddily.

"Hi, Ashley. I don't have good news for you; I'm so sorry. Your test was negative today. I'm so sorry."

My world stopped. I looked at Josh in surprise as my mouth moved open and shut without saying anything a couple of times. I couldn't believe my ears. How could I not be pregnant?

"Oh... what, what was... what was my level?"

Silence, then, "less than one."

That couldn't be right. She had to be wrong.

I paused and then started again. "Because I've been peeing on home pregnancy tests and have been getting positive pregnancy tests all week..."

"Well, that's probably from the trigger shot... oh no, you didn't have a trigger shot, did you? This was a frozen cycle... um. I'm not sure. But, I mean, it's totally negative today."

"Oh... okay."

"Yeah, I'm sorry. We'll have you stop your medications." I choked on a sob that had her pausing. "I'm not sure why those would come out positive because you didn't get hCG."

"Yeah, no. It's been positive since Monday. I tried all the tests: red line, blue line, digital, rapid, and early detection. Yeah..." I wiped my cheeks again.

"We recommend you stop the medication and then give the nurses a call. We won't have a chance to review your case until Wednesday. We can discuss your next steps after that." She paused briefly. "Do you have any more embryos?"

"We have two more that are frozen." I choked out through my clogged voice.

"Oh, you do!" Her voice picked up. "That's good. This time we can see if there's anything different we can do. Again, I'm so sorry."

"Alright, umm, thank you." At this point, I was barely holding it together.

We said our goodbyes and I took a shaky breath and tossed my phone toward our feet on the bed. I looked at Josh, at a loss for words. With tears in his eyes, he put down his phone that was still recording and said, "Come here, sweetie."

My head slammed into his chest, and the sobs came. We cried together and wondered what this meant. We knew IVF wasn't guaranteed, but when they originally said that Josh was the problem, a part of me assumed that the hardest part would be fertilizing the eggs. I figured once the eggs were fertilized, my uterus, which had no problems to date, besides being a fickle bitch, would accept the embryo and then move on. It didn't occur to me that my uterus wouldn't accept the healthy embryos.

I was more like Monica from *Friends* than I thought.

After we processed our emotions, we rallied and tried to talk it out. We were in disbelief. How could I not be pregnant? I was testing positive at home with urine tests, so why would a blood test show that I wasn't? Josh grabbed his phone and pulled up his Internet browser. He searched for reasons why. None of the results were good.

Apparently, if you have positive urine tests but negative blood tests, it can be a sign that you have cancer. So go figure.

But even so, I was still convinced I was pregnant. Even though she told me to stop the drugs, that my blood work results were zero and that there was absolutely no way I was pregnant. I just couldn't wrap my head around it. I just didn't believe her. I couldn't. There was no way that I couldn't be pregnant. I felt pregnant. Finally! And now she was telling me I wasn't?

This couldn't be right. I refused to believe it.

Maybe I was being delusional (the delusional never think they're delusional, I'm sure), but I just didn't believe our results.

After discussing it more with Josh, I called the clinic back on their after-hours line and asked the nurses and staff on call to call back immediately. In the meantime, Josh suggested I pee on another pregnancy test to see if the line had become fainter.

Even though, even if it was a chemical pregnancy (which meant that the embryo was implanted for only a short period and then aborted), the blood test would have tested the same as the pee test. The blood tests are so much more accurate. They should have been the same!

None of this made any sense!

And sure enough, two dark pink lines.

According to my blood hCG, I was definitely pregnant.

As we waited for the doctor to call me back, Josh and I kept searching for reasons why the blood test would be negative, but the urine test would be positive. It was all mostly the same answer every time. It indicated cancer.

Why not? I thought sourly. My faith in the universe wasn't super strong at this point, and the bitterness was overflowing. People had it much worse than poor, little, ole' me-but the anger wasn't letting me put that into perspective quite yet.

Josh asked me to go back through our timeline from the transfer on. I had a notebook of all my symptoms and each pregnancy test was dated and saved. (Hey, when you've been trying for years and finally get a real positive, you don't throw that puppy away!)

We compared the lines and how they progressively got darker.

We discussed my symptoms, which were more or less the same ones as previous transfers, which are all side effects of estrogen and progesterone. So those were almost nonfactors to consider. The one thing that stood out was a new, weird symptom. A few days after this transfer, I randomly got short of breath and had random heart palpitations. They were completely random: when I was driving my car, when I was eating dinner, when I was taking a shower, etc. There was no rhyme or reason to why I was getting heart palpitations. I just assumed because this was a new symptom, that this was an indicator of being pregnant.

So.

Walks like a duck quacks like a duck... Again, you know the saying.

When the doctor called us back, I could hear in her voice that she had done this a time or two. She was used to having this second conversation with desperate would-be parents. The type of parents that just couldn't understand why they weren't pregnant once again. And the second call back to affirm that the cycle did indeed fail. She seemed caring but very firm.

But that wasn't the case for us. I was pregnant. I knew I was. Something was wrong with the blood work.

"Ashley?"

"Yes, hi." I stumbled. "My husband encouraged me to call to clarify my thought process here. So, I mean, I just peed on another home pregnancy test two minutes ago, and it was strongly positive again. So, I just want to know. I know it's probably not likely, but is there any chance that my bloodwork was wrong?"

"I mean," she sighed like I was this pitiful, desperate thing. "I guess the chance is always there. So, if you want to come back tomorrow and have it done again, that's fine. I'm not quite sure why your result is coming out like that. All I can tell you is the report that I got. So you're more than welcome to come back tomorrow."

I stuck with it. "I didn't take a trigger shot or anything, so I shouldn't be testing positive if I wasn't positive."

"What's your diagnosis? Do you have PCOS?"

"No, just unexplained infertility at this point."

"Hmm, that is strange. That is very strange." A half-chuckle. "I could be wrong. I hope I'm wrong."

"So we had the transfer Friday, and I caved on Monday and tested. Which was a negative."

"Well, first thing, that is entirely too early to test..."

"Oh, absolutely. I know that and agree. I just couldn't help myself." I smiled weakly at Josh. "But then I tested again on Tuesday and got a faint positive. And again on Wednesday. And Thursday was darker. And I took multiple tests on Friday and Saturday, and the results were clearly there. Why else would I have hCG in my system if I wasn't pregnant? Is something wrong with me if it's not pregnancy?"

A pause. "I don't know. I can't say for sure. I don't have your chart in front of me. So I can't answer that for you. It's highly unusual, but certainly... if you want to come back in tomorrow for confirmation, that's the only thing I can offer."

I looked at Josh, and he nodded in agreement.

"Should we see someone when we come in? Or just do the bloodwork again?"

"Just talk to our nurses in the morning and tell them that you spoke to me. Tell them that because of the discrepancy, I told you to come back in."

"Has that ever happened before? That the blood test has shown negative, but urine tests are positive?" Josh chimed into the speakerphone.

"Yeah... It's very, very, very unusual." The doubt in her voice was almost tangible. "But call us in the morning. We'll fax over an order to your local hospital, so you don't have to drive down here, and we'll go from there. Don't stop your meds."

"Sounds like a plan." I agreed.

I could almost hear the faint sound of God laughing.

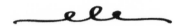

For the Super Bowl, I was a zombie. I felt like I was living through a haze and couldn't understand what had happened. I sat there in my Patriots paraphernalia, watching the game, but I just couldn't get into it. My head was one million miles away. I couldn't stop thinking about the blood work results and how they just couldn't be right. We were certain the hospital was wrong and agreed that I shouldn't stop the hormones because if I did, then we would lose our little embryo.

The next morning, we emailed our bosses and said something came up and that we'd both be in late. We sat around, waiting for the IVF nurses to call us back with the go-ahead that we could head into the lab. Given the distance, we didn't want to leave before they confirmed just in case they asked us to come in for a different time.

My phone started ringing shortly after eight. Josh and I started packing up while I answered.

I plopped down next to him on the couch, where he was loading his laptop and paperwork into his work backpack.

"Hi, Ashley?"

"Hi, yup, that's me." I half-smiled over at Josh and put the phone on speaker.

"Hi, this is Denise from the IVF team. I'm calling because I got your message about wanting to do more bloodwork?"

"Yes. We think the blood test results were wrong somehow or got mixed up. We want to come back and get my blood redrawn."

A pause.

"I don't understand... Why do you want to retest, honey? Your beta is positive."

Another pause.

Another heartbeat.

Josh and I looked at each other in shock.

I croaked out a rather crass, "are you fucking serious?"

Josh started crying across from me. I could feel my own throat start to close, my eyes burning. The relief was suffocating.

"Yeah, hun, your beta is at 147. Which is good. I don't know what the doctor was looking at, but you're definitely pregnant."

The world stopped spinning for just a split second.

Then it started again, and I felt *complete* for the first time in years.

I was pregnant.

Timeline

If you're a visual person, here's the timeline of events:

September 2013 – went off *The Pill*

May 2014 – graduated from master's program

Summer 2014 – finished all CPA exams

September 2014 – wedding

May 2015 – not preventing but not tracking/trying either

September 2015 – actively trying and tracking

March 2016 - laid off

August 2016 - coaching and new job

Fall/Winter 2016 - started tests

November 2016 - ultrasound

November 2016 - follow-up - high prolactin

November 2016 - endocrinology for Prolactinoma (brain tumor)

December 2016 - brain MRI and HSG

December 2016 – HSG

January 2017 - progesterone bloodwork

January 2017 - last apt with Bradlee - sent to McBride

February 2017 -Josh sees first urologist

March 2017 – Dr. McBride in VT

April 2017 - Josh sees Urologist in MA, twice

April 2017 – cystoscopy

April 2017 – sent back to McBride

April 2017 – Referred to IVF Clinic #1 to IVF to start in May

May 2017 – Week before we start, the IVF clinic closes

May 2017 – Find new IVF clinic

May 24, 2017 - Orientation at IVF Clinic #2 (referred to as Burr Medical)

May 2017– first apt at Burr Medical

May/June 2017 – Moved to hourly

June 2017 – receive drugs

July 2017 – insurance debacle

July 15, 2017 – retrieval

July 2017 - PGS testing. Four surviving embryos

August 2017 – first transfer

August 2017 – TWW and bloodwork

September 2017 – bloodwork and ultrasound – lining was okay

September 2017 – second transfer

September 2017 – Spotting 3 days after transfer. Heavy brown bleeding a week after transfer.

September 29, 2017 – phone call regarding my care plan. Possible chronic endometritis

October 2017 – Endometrial Biopsy

December 3, 2017 – Second retrieval

One surviving embryo

December 2017 – anesthesia to remove a polyp

January 2018 - start of my cycle

January 26, 2018 – transfer

February 4, 2018 – negative blood test phone call

February 5, 2018 – Life-changing phone call

About the Author

Guion was born and raised in New Hampshire and never wants to leave. Married to her high-school sweetheart, they never expected the rollercoaster of infertility to darken their doorstep. She felt overwhelmingly alone during their infertility process, and so she hopes her story spreads awareness to others.

She read once that one in seven couples experience infertility.

So *you* (whoever *you* are) are not alone.

Find your people – in person or online. And get that support system in place.

You're going to want them!

Guion is the storyteller in their house, and her two young boys demand new ones every night. In 2021, she finally put pen to paper (or fingers to keys) and decided to share them with others in her **Bugaboo Creek Day School** stories collection (see titles at the end of this book).

Social Media Information

DID YOU ENJOY THIS book? If so, please visit **www.alguion.com** and sign up for the newsletter to receive additional scenes, freebies, and updates on future releases.

Also, if this book brought you a smile, please review it on your purchasing platform (and copy it to Goodreads if you're willing and able). This helps to spread the word about the book. *Social proof to other readers is important.*

(image of our actual pregnancy announcement photo)

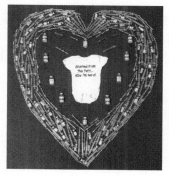

OTHER BOOKS BY A. L. GUION

Children's picture books (intended age 2-5 years)
Bugaboo Creek Day School Series (available on all major platforms):

1. Hero Teacher Ted

2. Picking My Perfect Pet

3. Mia's Potty Practice

4. Super Feelings

5. Try Again, Tommy

6. Annie's Asthma Attack

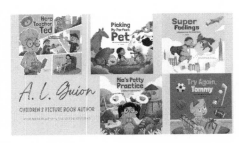

Life Lessons Series (available on all major platforms):
1. Going To The Dentist

Website: <u>www.alguion.com</u>

CHEAT SHEET FOR WELL-MEANING BUT IRRITATING FRIENDS AND FAMILY

PEOPLE AROUND YOU WILL say a variety of things that will rub you the wrong way. Here are a few we encountered that made this journey harder for us.

Feel free to print this list out and hand it over to people that you're planning on telling about your infertility struggles.

A better (more appropriate version without that top rant) is available for printing on my website (www.alguion.com)

DO NOT SAY:

- It will happen when it's supposed to

- You just need to relax, and it will happen

- Infertile person: "I'm tired," well-meaning person: "maybe you're pregnant!" (don't say this)

- God has a plan

- It will happen when the time is right, and maybe right now isn't the right time

- Just relax! It will happen!

- Maybe you aren't supposed to have kids

- There's a reason that an egg and a sperm won't fertilize and using science to force it isn't healthy.

- Stressing about it is only going to make it worse

- You'll understand when you have your own kid

- You're young. You have plenty of time

- Don't wait forever. You're not getting any younger

- No time is perfect. You just have to do it and make it work

- Your parents deserve to have some grandbabies. You've made them wait long enough.

- Trust me, wait to have kids. Travel and do all sorts of fun stuff because that goes out the window once you have kids.

- Enjoy sleeping through the night while you can.

- If you want a kid so bad, take one of mine.

- Did you see that so-and-so just announced she was pregnant?

- My cousin's college roommate has a friend that has a sister that tried for years to get pregnant and got pregnant once she stopped trying. And that was after six failed IVF cycles!

- Well, trying is the fun part!

- Are you tracking your cycles?

- Have you tried....

- Just do IVF...

- You think life is expensive now? Wait till you have a kid! (Right, like fertility treatments are free...)

- **Just have sex! ;-)**

The most important thing to a couple trying to conceive (at least for Josh and me) was to feel supported. We don't want stories about success or failures, we don't want your opinion or suggestions, and we don't want you to solve our problems because we already have a team of licensed medical professionals trying to do just that! We want you to sit there, listen to our struggles, offer support (do not minimize the struggles or our feelings), and just be a sympathetic ear. Do NOT say that IVF (or something else) isn't that bad – one: it's condescending; two: YOU pump your body full of hormones and say it doesn't take a toll; three: that shit is expensive, and four: it's still not even guaranteed to work! Which is a HUGE misconception. The odds of getting pregnant via IVF are not certain, so do not even imply it.

Just listen. That's all we want. And don't hate us if we stop "liking" all your baby photos.
You have no idea how hard this is.

Made in United States
Troutdale, OR
09/21/2023

13094771R20152